DONE WITH BEING FAT

By
T.C. Hale & Others

Cover Designed by Tony Hale & Gabe Evans; Nuts photos courtesy of Craig Barnes Photography

File Version 2.2.1

For Mom, if only someone had taught me this earlier.

WHAT THE CELEBRITIES SAY

"Working with Tony is like jumping into the arms of your favorite aunt. Except it's not. At all. I mean, his methods work. But it's not like that at all." - **Jane Lynch (*Glee*)**

"I confess to being a full-blown 'gymophobe.' (I still have flashbacks of my mean fourth-grade gym teacher!) Tony actually makes the gym panic-attack free." - **Tom Kenny (Voice of Spongebob)**

"Wait. You mean the short skinny trainer dude with the neon sneakers who writes books about women's menstrual cramps? Did he ever get a single menstrual cramp? I don't think so. The guy who helps fat people get skinnier? Was he ever fat ? I don't think so. And what's with the whole fake I don't talk thing? Is it turrets? If he did talk, would it be a string of expletives even I would be offended by? I guess he has a sense of humor. That's something good." - **Betty Thomas (Director: 28 *Days*, *The Brady Bunch Movie*, etc.)**

"You can argue with Tony, or you can do what he says and buy smaller jeans." - **Kari Wahlgren (Voice of Tigress, *Kung Fu Panda: Legends of Awesomeness*)**

"Tony took on my Jewish-Cuban hips and he won! He let me pretend the punching bag was my ex's mom. That was fun and I got in shape too. I adore him but my tush loves him more." - **Brigitte Bako (*G Spot*, *The Red Shoe Diaries*)**

"I always look forward to my weekly beatings from Tony." - **Tucker Barkley (Dance Choreographer: *The X Factor*)**

"So you know that moment when you are just finishing a hard workout with Tony and he says, 'Alright, you warmed up? We can start now?' and then he laughs... I hate that moment." - **Kayla Radomski (*So You Think You Can Dance*)**

Acknowledgements

Thank you to my co-authors and collaborators. Without your help and patience, this book would still be a big stack of ideas.

Special thanks to Sarah Griswold, for rewriting nearly every word of this book in the hopes of making me sound less stupid. It's fun to be able to say I wrote a book, even though meximelt and Fonzie are the only two words remaining from my original manuscript.

Thank you to my readers, editors and contributors: Sam Bangs, Alex and Red Donnally, and Silena Smith-Shamey.

Thank you to my brother, Richard, who is also an author, for his insight into how to not be a sucky author. I don't understand why you haven't checked out his books yet. He writes great thrillers.

www.RichardCHaleAuthor.com

Finally, I'd like to thank you, the reader, for allowing me to entertain myself throughout this book, instead of just getting to the point, even though you may want to lose weight right now. I thank you for indulging me.

DISCLAIMER

This book is not intended as a substitute for the medical recommendations of a physician or other healthcare provider. Don't be stupid. It's just a book. This book is intended to entertain and to offer information to help the reader cooperate with physicians and health professionals in a mutual quest of improved well-being.

The identities of people described in this book have been changed to protect confidentiality.

The *Done With That* series is written and published as an information resource and educational guide for both professionals and non-professionals. It should not be used to replace medical advice.

The publisher and the author are not responsible for any goods and/or services offered or referred to in this book and expressly disclaim all liability in connection with the fulfillment of orders for any such goods and/or services and for any damages, loss, or expense to person or property arising out of or relating to them. You are responsible for your own health and wellness.

PLEASE VISIT THE AUTHOR'S WEBSITE AT:

www.DoneWithThatBooks.com

Or follow him on Twitter and Facebook:

www.twitter.com/KickItInTheNuts

www.facebook.com/KickItInTheNuts

Table of Contents

INTRODUCTION

About The Authors

Geez. Where do I start? My name is Tony Hale. I use the pen name "T.C. Hale" because if you Google "Tony Hale" you find four hundred thousand pictures of Buster Bluth from *Arrested Development*. If you're unfamiliar with the actor, one of his first big national spots was that Volkswagen commercial with the guy doing the robot in his car. I can remember studying at The Groundlings (an Improv school that churns out a lot of *SNL* players) when a girl in my class told me that her friend's name was Tony Hale too, and that he was the guy in the Volkswagen commercial. I recall thinking, "That guy's going to call dibs on my name before I do," and that's pretty much how it worked out. I run into Tony around town from time to time and he's actually a super nice guy. The first time I met him, he was shopping at Whole Foods. I walked up to him, didn't say a word, and just handed him my driver's license. "No way!" he said after seeing my name.

Turns out, he was excited to meet me because he had heard of my existence since I have an acting credit that is listed on his IMDb.com page. When I was touring as a comic, I was dating a girl who booked one of the leads in an independent film called *Raging Hormones*. Visiting her on set, the director asked me to drive by in a scene and make fun of the main character. It earned me a film credit, but they attached it to the wrong Tony Hale. Since this was literally THE worst movie that has ever been created, I decided to let Tony keep the credit. Tony told me that he always wondered if that was a real movie and how it got on his resume. I let him know that he should be proud to have been involved in a film that was even more brilliant than *Gigli*. But, enough about my name already. What about the rest? How did I get here?

I guess like most natural health and nutrition researchers, my background comes from a professional career in stand-up comedy. I found that, as I traveled across the country from city-to-city, if I had a show that didn't go well, I figured that town must be constipated. With the realization that very few things are ever funny when you can't poop, I began using science in my comedy career. Handing out laxatives at my show seemed odd at first... Um, I think that's as far as I can BS my way through that story. That's really not how it happened at all and I apologize for lying so early in our relationship. The truth is, yes, I toured as a comic, but the only thing I learned about natural health on the road was that, in the towns where people drank a lot of alcohol, their bodies were a lot fatter and I was a lot funnier.

I became a natural health and nutrition researcher by necessity. On Valentine's Day 2004, I took my girlfriend at the time to see The Dan Band at the club, Hollywood and Highland. Most of the night, I talked over the loud music. The next day, my voice was gone and it didn't come back. Over the next year or so, 23 doctors, specialists, and surgeons couldn't figure out what the problem was. With each doctor and each medication, my health seemed to decline a little more. After exhausting my way through doctors, speech therapists, natural practitioners, and a six-figure accumulation of expenses, I told everybody to piss off and decided I was going to figure this out myself.

And that's what I did. Over the next six years I did nothing but read books, research nutrition experts, and attend workshops and seminars across the country. As I searched for my own answers, I kept stumbling across answers to problems that my friends were dealing with. I was so amazed to find explanations that I had never heard of that I started to share them with my friends. When I emailed my buddy Greg and explained to him some of the underlying issues that can make a person have to sit on the toilet twelve times a day, he ran some measurements on himself to see what the likely causes were and his chemistry matched up perfectly with most people who have similar issues. He tried the things I showed him and he was able to poop like a normal human, once or twice a day, instead of shooting soup out the back door all day.

As one friend would tell another friend, people kept emailing me and asking if I could help them understand their health issues. But I was working as a personal trainer and didn't have time to teach all those people how to look at their own chemistry to understand why they're dealing with what they're dealing with. That is, until a guy named Jim, who was so impressed with how I taught his friend how to understand and improve his insomnia, offered me $500 to help him, too. That's when I realized, "Oh, this is a business." After all, I would have gladly paid someone $10,000 to help me correct my issue years earlier. That's a lot of money, but it still would have saved me $90,000 and reduced the six years it took for me to start getting my voice back. With this revelation, I started a career as a health coach. I've never advertised, but today I help some of the biggest stars and most influential people in the entertainment industry better understand how they can use nutrition to improve their health. That is also what I'm going to do with you in these pages. Isn't that nice of me? You don't even have your own show and I'm still going to help you.

Before you look at anything I have to say as gospel, I want to make sure that I am very clear on the fact that I am not a doctor and I don't claim to be any sort of doctor or licensed professional. I don't even watch *House*. I used to think M*A*S*H was funny, but that hardly makes me a doctor. What I am is a guy who became fed up with the system and decided I would find my answers elsewhere. I'm just a guy who had no choice but to keep digging until solutions were uncovered. I had no choice because it was becoming clear that I wasn't going to be able to talk again unless I found real answers. If it were anything else, I probably would have given up after two years. For example, if I were just walking with a limp, or I couldn't talk without whistling and spitting on people, or whatever the case may be, I probably would have just learned to live with it. But since I was very determined to get my voice back, I was willing to do the work. Remember, a stand-up comic with no voice is just a mime—and I can't imagine anyone becomes a mime by choice.

So, if you're looking for credentials, buy another book. I encountered plenty of professionals with credentials, certifications, licenses, awards, accolades, expensive offices... you name it. One guy even had a live ostrich that lived in the backyard of his office complex. (That didn't help, either.) The professionals I consulted had it all. Yet, none of them could help me. As a result of that experience, I find that I'm more interested in the truth than I am in credentials. Over the last 60 years, doctor after doctor who went outside the box to try to truly help patients (by working to correct the actual causes of their illnesses instead of just treating symptoms) have been stripped of their licenses, discredited, and basically run out of town. Sadly, this happens frequently. It seems like every time someone makes a significant splash in the mainstream market with any advances that could help people correct health issues naturally, that individual is discredited so that the masses will go back to spending billions on drugs that only mask their symptoms.

With these *Done With That* books, since my co-authors and I know this information will spread fast, we're going to go another route. After all, when people finally get answers to problems they have been dealing with for decades, they talk about it. So we're setting up a system where people can learn about their body without having that system discredited. It can't be discredited because I am the voice and I'm telling you right now, I HAVE NO CREDENTIALS. I'm just a schmuck comedian and personal trainer who was willing to dig for his own answers. And now I'm sharing what I've learned with you, so you can dig for your answers a little quicker. Am I a doctor? No. Do I have a license? Heck no. Do we really need one more person following the same system that isn't working? I don't even shave every day, I've filed for bankruptcy in my life, I don't understand what color shirt I'm allowed to wear with brown pants, and I'm writing this book in my boxers. Does that sound like somebody who has credentials?

Though I am not the only author in this series of books, I have been elected to be the voice and will be the only known author for many of our titles. In this book, as well as others in this series, my co-authors and contributors are made up of doctors, M.D.s, medical and natural health researchers, and some of the most well respected educators who teach doctors from all over the world about nutrition. When I traveled the country looking for answers, I found a number of individuals who have dedicated their lives to this work. I've approached many of them to help me in this effort. Though some have chosen to have their names added as co-authors to a number of our titles, many are keeping their identity anonymous, so as to protect their practices and keep the powers-that-be from trying to discredit the amazing work they are doing.

Although I won't be sharing the names of most of my co-authors with you, I will share the pioneers from the 1930s and 1940s who first discovered these truths. That was the one constant that I seemed to find no matter who I talked to. Most of the experts I found had studied doctors from the 30s, 40s and 50s, back when a doctor was allowed to think. I'll talk about the work of these pioneers throughout our time together, and I'll even point you in the direction of some of their amazing books so you can dig deeper if you find this information as interesting as I did.

Odds are someone who experienced incredible results recommended this book to you. So, my suggestion is for you to put your trust in the experience of your friend instead of the authorities that seem to be more interested in profit than results. After all, wasn't it Benjamin Franklin who once said, "Though I have welcomed the words from authorities my whole life, it might be time for them to go flog themselves," or something like that?

CHAPTER ONE

Hi

How close are you to completely snapping? Count your calories, watch your portions, don't eat fast food, go vegan, eliminate gluten, eat only raw foods, go on a juice fast, avoid red meat, wear a vibrating belt around your waist all day, eat what you want unless it has flavor, walk northeast for 30 minutes after dinner. Is there a limit to the bad advice you can receive before you scream? As annoying as it is to hear such a wide variety of suggestions, odds are, you've probably tried some of these methods. Or do you find that you've been more attracted to the Hollywood grapefruit cleanse, "only eat things you find in your couch cushions," or ice cream sandwich diet-type programs?

Maybe you've bought into the whole "just burn more calories than you consume" camp, or maybe you feel like you could finally lose the weight if you could just find time to work out an extra 15 hours a week. Maybe you're here because you're an infomercial junkie. Maybe you spend less money on actual food than you spend on blenders, juicers, DVDs, and other contraptions.

It's time to step away from your maple syrup / cayenne pepper / lemon juice concoction and learn the truth about weight loss, body fat, and even more importantly, being a healthy human. For some people, just improving their health can allow fat to fall off. But this book is not about helping SOME people. This book is about teaching you how to look at your own body and find appropriate solutions for you—not just the popular solution, *your* solution.

There are reasons why some people can watch an ice cream commercial and gain weight, while others can work at Ben & Jerry's, get paid only in ice cream, and never gain an ounce. These are the same scientific reasons that allowed your friend to lose weight on the exact diet that caused you to pack on twenty pounds.

If you're extremely overweight, or even if you just can't seem to knock off that last five pounds, my co-authors and I will help you understand some of the actual causes behind your weight gain and teach you how other people have been correcting those causes for years. People all over the world are learning how they can look at their own physiology and understand their biological individuality. These people are learning about nutritional and lifestyle changes, specific to their body, that can help them lose weight and keep it off. And they're doing it without the help of surgical procedures or medications.

Since it is widely accepted that people can have "bad genes" or a slow metabolism, and that's just the way it is, I find that my clients are always surprised when they find answers to questions like:

- How can I figure out which food choices are best for me?
- How can I lose the weight and keep it off?
- Why do I crave so much junk?
- Why is the public so misguided about weight loss?
- How did I get so fat?
- Why do so many people that resort to weight loss surgeries end up gaining all of their weight back?

My co-authors and I agree that, for the most part, the common answers to these questions are all over the map. I wonder if there will ever be another topic where so many people feel like they have the answer. The reality is this: It's not that nobody has the right answers, it's that nobody is asking the right questions. Not that I've fully examined every diet out there—I doubt that would even be humanly possible—but it is my experience that every diet on the planet can work... for SOMEBODY. However, no diet will work for EVERYBODY.

The problem with most diets today is that they are a one-size-fits-all approach. Sure, there are diets that are specific to blood type, or specific to symptoms or conditions; but nobody looks at individuals and how they are processing different foods, or even how their bodies are operating. I know you've heard the media say that obesity is a condition or even a disease, but it's not. Excess body fat is a symptom created by malfunctions in the body or by the operator of that body. In the world of weight loss, the popular approach is to attack that symptom.

The same holds true for any topic on health. A person is branded by symptoms. Do shoes come only in one size? How about bras or even contact lenses? No. We look at people as individuals for just about anything they need, except their health. In the world of healthcare, we're a one-trick pony. We're like a 7-11 that sells only Skittles. We look only at the symptoms instead of looking at the person who is suffering from the symptoms. And when our great, great grandkids learn about our health care system in their history classes, they will laugh at us. They will point, and they will laugh... and our only excuse will be that the characters on *Grey's Anatomy* were so dreamy, we just believed everything they said.

Done With Being Fat was written to help you look at your own biological identity, understand how your specific body is operating, and make the necessary changes to help your body function in a more optimal way... so you can fit back into your favorite jeans without needing a shoe horn.

Slackers, Whack-Jobs, and Geniuses

Everyone is invited to join in. You're going to have the chance to decide what you want to get out of this book. You'll have the opportunity to begin implementing what you learn from the very beginning. Some of you will discover life-changing information and learn how to implement that knowledge within the first few chapters. You may be able to reach your goals using what you've learned without ever reading past chapter six.

Though the first six chapters will likely provide information you've never heard before, many of you will want to continue reading. Maybe you tend to become a total nut-job every time you start a new diet. The goal will be to set yourself up for weight loss, while still providing your body with everything it needs to function as a reasonable human being. Admit it; some diets have made many of us quite the psycho.

Finally, I'd like to welcome any geniuses and those crazy people who read about something scientific and feel like they need to learn about every single aspect. That was me (the crazy person, not the genius). I became quite the researching maniac once I realized there were real answers out there. For you folks, I've included some pretty sciency stuff and I'll provide more in-depth explanations in the appendix section of the book. If you still want to learn more, you can also read my upcoming book, *Urine You're Out: Understanding Simple Biochemistry for Optimal Health*. That book goes into a lot more detail and was written for healthcare professionals or those who are very serious about learning how the body really works.

Not everybody wants to understand the science. It wouldn't be the first time someone has said to me, "Hey Monkey Boy, just tell me what to do and I'll do it." With that in mind, know that you will have the choice of using the easy-to-follow methods in this book to reach your own goals, or you can dig into all aspects of this book and gain a new understanding about nutrition, the human body, and why health issues are so common today.

Why Am I Reading A Natural Health Book Written By A Comedian?

While working at a seafood restaurant as a teenager, I once found a nickel inside a raw oyster. A nickel! It was as if the oyster was saving up to buy a pearl because nobody told him he was supposed to make his own. Well, in the same way that you can find something beautiful—like a pearl—in something so gross and snot-looking—like an oyster—you can also find something unexpected—like a nickel. My point is, I was surprised to find cash inside an oyster, but I was still able to use the cash on my way home that night when I stopped by the Taco Bell drive-through. So, just because you find information on natural health in a place you might not expect, that doesn't mean it can't be useful to you. My nickel helped pay for a Meximelt with no pico sauce, which was very useful to me.

I studied nutrition for twenty years before I came across the information I am sharing with you in this book. I truly thought I knew what I was talking about when it came to weight loss, but since I had my own health issues that were plaguing me, I was forced to do a tremendous amount of research on my own and I was shocked at what I discovered. Now, you're about to benefit from my need to dig for real answers for myself.

As it turns out, many of the keys to health are also the keys to trimming your tummy, and vice versa.

About This Series Of Books

In the *Done With That* series of natural health books, I'll be helping you look at your health, body, and nutrition in a way that is different from any other natural health book you've ever read. Instead of just looking at a condition and talking about all the "natural remedies" that have been known to work for that condition, we're going to spend most of our time looking at YOU—the individual. Focusing only on the condition or symptoms is the biggest mistake in the world of health. It's like focusing on the straw that broke the camel's back instead of seeing the inordinate load that needs to be lifted off. With this series of books, it is my goal to offer you other options.

The truth is, every symptom or condition can have three or four different underlying causes. That's why so many "remedies" or methods will work great for one person with a particular symptom, but will make another person with the same symptom much worse. Nobody is looking at each individual and the actual cause of the symptom for *that* individual.

I placed a disclaimer at the beginning of this book stating that this information should not replace any medical advice, etc, etc. Let's look a little deeper into this topic so you can have an understanding of what you might get out of this book. I don't want you to look at this book like it's going to be a tool to "beat your fat." It's never a good idea to focus on trying to eliminate, declare war on, cure, or kick any problem. Once you see the direction this knowledge can take you, you will see that trying to "beat" something is very rarely successful. Instead, the goal here is to teach you about the body's operational systems and what imbalances might be pushing in the wrong direction when common symptoms, like weight gain, show up. Then I'm going to show you steps that others have taken in order to move their bodies back to a more balanced operational state. If you understand this objective, you will see that the goal should be to move toward health instead of trying to escape from, or beat down, symptoms or "disease."

Look at it this way... if you're in a dark, locked closet, there is nothing but darkness. You can't destroy the darkness. You can't beat it down or even run from it. To put your effort into changing that darkness into something else would be very frustrating and time consuming and your friends would say, "Hey, you've been in that closet for a long time... what the heck are you doing in there?" But if you turn on a light, the darkness will disappear on its own. Darkness cannot exist in a place where there is light. You didn't have to do anything to convince the darkness to leave or to stop tormenting you, you just invited something else into the closet that made it impossible for the darkness to exist there. You invited in the light and the darkness went away on its own.

If you have read any of my other *Done With That* titles, or even my more comical *Kick It in the Nuts* books, some content of this book (as well as some of the jokes) may sound familiar to you. Much of this book will teach you how to look at you and your chemistry. Knowing your own chemistry is the most important factor when dealing with any health issue. In each title, I have given readers a foundation of information about chemical imbalances in the body, how to test their own chemistry, and how to view the information they find through testing. Those tools and methods never change no matter what health issue you would like to see improve. If you already have a good understanding of those techniques from one of my other books, you'll be miles ahead and you will be able to use this title to better understand how specific imbalances can relate to weight gain.

Take The Quiz

If you have not already taken this quiz online or had a friend email it to you, take the time to answer these ten questions now. If you answer YES to any of the following questions, acquiring information about your body's biological individuality could be life-transforming. If you answer YES to many or most of the following questions, you might want to carry this book with you wherever you go—at least until you can answer NO to most of them. Many of the topics covered in this quiz are experienced by a large percentage of the population and these people walk through life believing this is just the way it is. By the time you finish this book, you will know that is not the case. You will know that the issues below can see improvement in almost any individual who is willing to put forth the effort. Good luck on your quiz, I know I didn't really let you prepare in any way. I always hated the teacher that would pull stunts like that.

(1) Do cravings frequently derail your weight loss attempts?
    YES NO
(2) Have you ever used a diet that worked for others, yet you saw no real results?
    YES NO
(3) Do you frequently pass gas after meals?
    YES NO
(4) Do you often burp after meals or feel bloated? (Even just small burps.)
    YES NO
(5) Does your meal ever feel like it's sitting in your stomach like a rock for too long?
    YES NO
(6) Have you ever lost weight on a diet, only to gain it all back, and more?
    YES NO
(7) Do you crave sweet or salty foods?
    YES NO
(8) Do some foods make you nauseous?
    YES NO
(9) Is your stool sometimes lighter than the color of corrugated cardboard?
    YES NO
(10) Do you turn into a werewolf or become some other type of unreasonable creature if you go too long without eating?
    YES NO

How did you do? If you can answer no to all of those questions, you may qualify to read this book for the jokes and then pass it along to a friend. But if you answered yes to one or more of those questions, you will likely have some life-long mysteries solved for yourself by the time you get to chapter six. That's a pretty fun reward considering you just failed the first pop quiz you've had since the tenth grade.

A New Light On Health

Let's get started by putting down a foundation. That foundation is to answer the questions that will run through your head for the duration of this book. "Why have I never heard this stuff? Why didn't my doctor tell me this when he pointed out that I had gained so much weight that I now have cankles? Is nothing in this book true or does my doctor hate me?"

While digging for answers, there was one topic that really changed the way I looked at my health, the choices I was making, and where I wanted to find help. Before I explain this, I just want to be clear that in no way am I saying that the entire medical world is a shot in the dark, or that the entire system is more evil than that blonde guy from *The Karate Kid*. The advances and information that medical professionals and researchers have provided are truly amazing and many of them do indeed save and/or prolong lives. Even some medications that result in horrible side effects still provide you with the ability to buy yourself some time and fight off a certain death long enough to really improve your health or correct the underlying problem. The only knock on how the whole system works that I cover here is this: We are given only half the story.

With that in mind, here's the piece of information I came across again and again while I was trying to figure out why each doctor and each medication was making me worse instead of better. This is the piece of information that woke me up to the realization that it was time to put my health back into my own hands. Not that I didn't still need help from health professionals, but that I would become a player in the process of understanding what my options really were and what would be best for me. Here it is: *The vast majority of curricula that are taught in medical schools in this country were put together by organizations that were founded by, or are funded by, pharmaceutical companies.* Read that again.

So let me get this straight… The people who make the most money from our being sick are the same people who are teaching our doctors how to make us healthy? I need you to stop and think about that for just a second with the intelligent part of your brain—not the part that just listens to what we're taught, or to what the media or our friends say, and simply accepts it.

How Medications Work

Before I talk about how medications work, please make sure you understand that in no way am I suggesting you stop taking any medications you are currently using. In most cases, medication is doing a job, and the person taking it needs that medication to continue doing its job, so just chucking it in the trash could be dangerous for some people. But once you begin to understand why you're likely dealing with the issues that you're dealing with, and how some people improve them by making better choices and moving body chemistry in the right direction, then you can decide for yourself if you want to accomplish that. Once you improve an issue by making more ideal decisions, you can then discuss with your doctor the possibility of reducing, or removing, the need for any meds. But promise me you won't try to do this on your own because that's just dumb. If you're currently on any meds, chances are great that you are going to need help from a professional, and the knowledge you receive in this book will be a great starting point to help you make better choices and communicate more effectively with that professional.

Here's how most medications work. Nearly all medications are synthetic, man-made substances; otherwise the manufacturer couldn't patent the drugs and make billions because it's not legal to patent a natural substance. However, most synthetic substances that enter the body will be filtered out by the liver and removed. That's the liver's job. So, if you put a drug in, the liver will filter it out and the drug won't be able to stay in the body and fulfill its purpose, rendering it worthless. To correct this, manufacturers upped the dosages in drugs to overwhelm the liver so enough of the drug can stay in your system and do the job (or give a physiological reaction) as it is intended to do. Well guess what? It works. The liver can't remove all of it and the drug often corrects the symptom it was intended to correct. Yet it does so at the cost of punching your liver in the mouth with every dose. Not only can this eventually lead to liver damage (which is why nearly every drug commercial states something along the lines of, "not to be used by those with liver disease"), but even in the first dose the drug is overwhelming the liver and restricting the liver from doing the job it was intended to do: Removing foreign and toxic substances. As the liver gets backed up and can't remove enough junk, the body will often store this junk in fat cells, or deposit it into joints and tissues.

Think of it like that episode of *I Love Lucy* when Lucy is working in the chocolate factory on the conveyor belt. As the chocolate starts to come in faster than she has the ability to keep up, she starts to cram the chocolate in her mouth, pockets, hat, anywhere she can find a safe place. If the body left junk in your bloodstream, it could disrupt the delicate balance and you could literally die. Since the balance of the bloodstream is so important, the body wouldn't let that extreme imbalance happen so it just stores bad stuff in fat cells or other tissues and plans on coming back later to remove it when the coast is clear. Unfortunately, with our taking medications consistently and constantly punching our liver in the mouth, along with all the junk we put in our bodies, the coast is never clear and we can begin to swell like the Stay Puft Marshmallow Man as we accumulate stored water, fat or toxicity in places where it should not be. So, when we gain weight, it is actually our body's way of saving our life. Now, weight gain does have its own health dangers when it becomes excessive, but isn't it smarter for the body to gain weight until the excess weight causes a problem over the choice of dying this Thursday because of all the toxins left in the bloodstream? This is only one possible cause for weight gain. I go over many more possibilities in this book, so keep reading. You can also watch video clips from my documentary, *Why Am I So Fat?*, at www.WhyAmISoFatMovie.com. This film will be released in 2013.

To share more information on medications and how the medical world operates, I wrote a chapter that includes more thoughts and funny stories on how the medical world operates (some were a little too funny for this book) and you can read it at: www.DoneWithThatBooks.com. I feel this info should be shared with everyone for free so I added this chapter to my website instead of putting it in my books. Just click on "Hidden Chapter." It has even been set-up so you can email this "Hidden Chapter" to a friend for free.

How To Use This Book

There are a number of factors that can cause weight gain and those reasons truly are different for everyone. To give a high percentage of readers an opportunity to start seeing improvements right away, I have ordered the chapters according to their priority, in my opinion. Each chapter covers a topic, or group of ideas, so that you can move through one chapter at a time and implement what you learn as you go. You may find that some chapters don't apply to you at all. Keep in mind, topics I placed at the beginning of the book are there for a reason. The early chapters cover the problems that need to be addressed in one way or another by most people dealing with weight issues.

The final appendix section holds all the advanced, geeky stuff for those who really want to jump into the rabbit hole.

We're all walking around in these bodies that are pretty much the most amazing mechanisms on the planet, yet we hardly know how the human body works. Pharmaceutical companies bombard us with so many ads that we all feel like we're dying before we're thirty. Ads like, "Do you have hair growing out of the top of your head? Have you ever sneezed? Click here to find out if you may be at risk for face cancer." A freaked-out public is a public that spends money in fear. Education about how your body functions can relieve fears.

Testing Tools You'll Need For This Book

In chapter seven, I dig in to simple self-testing and how to look at your own chemistry and get a picture of how your body is operating. Before you get to that, I want to touch on some tools that will be helpful so you can get a hold of them before you get to that section of the book. These tools can normally be found and ordered on the website, www.NaturalReference.com, but can also be found at just about any drug store and/or health food store in your area. I had such a hard time finding the tools and supplements that are effective that I partnered with an online store so I could tell them exactly what needed to be made available to the public. You'll be able to find most of the tools I talk about on the Natural Reference website.

pH Testing Strips

Some drug stores carry these and most health food stores keep them in stock. Just don't let them sell you other "alkalizing" products when they see you picking up pH testing strips. There is a LOT of bad information out there about pHs, so don't waste your time on that frontier like I did. You'll learn the truth about pHs later in this book. A package or roll of pH strips will usually run between $10-18. Health store clerks also sell a lot of ketone strips to those on the Atkins Diet so be sure they don't send you home with ketone strips when you ask for pH strips.

Blood Pressure Cuff

This is a pretty important tool if you're overweight, and one I would recommend buying. The money you spend will be well worth having the ability to monitor your progress. You can get a good one for around $50. Many of you won't know if you're on the right track without one. I like the push-button style that does all the work for you and has a cuff that is easy to put on yourself. You can look at the styles on www.NaturalReference.com to see examples of acceptable units. It usually does not matter which one you get, as long as you have a way to see if you're improving or if you need to make adjustments. You can also buy the arm wrap in different sizes if your weight has greatly increased the size of your arms. The wrist types are okay too, but generally not as accurate and seem to run a little low on the reading. Many drug stores also have those big sit-down machines that allow you to check your blood pressure while you're in the store. These are suitable if a blood pressure cuff is not in your budget, but it sure is nice to be able to check your blood pressure at home when you need to.

Stopwatch

You can also use a common digital kitchen timer or anything with a second hand. Or, I am also pretty sure there is an app for that.

Glucometer

This is a great tool to own and every household in the country should have one. The glucometer is sold separately from the glucometer testing strips because the strips expire, whereas the glucometer does not. You can find a glucometer pretty cheap these days, but the strips can cost around $50 for a pack of 50. If you have friends who are diabetic, ask them if you can use their glucometer one morning before you eat anything. If you find that your blood sugar is in a good range, you might be able to go without this tool for a while if you need to budget things out. However, if you are extremely overweight, I suggest investing in this tool from the get-go.

Wha'd He Say?

So far, you've learned:

- There is no diet that is right for every person.
- The people that profit the most from us being sick are the same people teaching our doctors how to keep us healthy.
- In order to get the most from this book, you need to acquire a few simple testing tools so you can look at your own chemistry and see how your body is operating.

CHAPTER TWO

What's With The Fat?

If you've been overweight for a while now, this book is probably not your first rodeo. I find that most of my overweight clients have made a minimum of ten different attempts to lose weight by the time they find me. You may have tried anything from counting calories, to having someone deliver meals to your doorstep every morning, to liquefying everything you eat in a $400 blender. Mmm, meatloaf shake. Once you understand the variety of problems that can create weight gain, I have a feeling you're going to be a little upset that nobody has supplied you with the information I'm about to share. I hope you're ready, because it's about to get jazzy.

What's Behind Body Fat?

Be mindful that just because an issue *can* create weight gain doesn't mean that it is the cause behind *your* weight gain. I feel that it is important for you to understand the causes behind the causes. Understanding will make it easier and more motivating to do the work to improve those underlying causes. Answers to your "whys" can also reduce anxiety and remove that "why does this happen to me?" feeling.

Stored body fat is often the result of a combination of circumstances and that combination can be different for each person. For example, chapter three talks about digestion and how this one factor is the most common underlying cause for weight gain—especially obesity. However, the reasons that a person may be having digestive issues, or how those issues are manifesting trouble in the body, can be different for each of us.

Some of the topics I cover you will have heard before. Some you may have instinctively believed to be true. And some will fully freak you out. In any case, know that you may have to re-learn concepts you believed to be true in the past. My question will be, did those concepts work for you? If they did, you would probably be reading a different book right now. Maybe that Tina Fey book? I hear it's funny.

Why Am I Getting Fat? My Friend Never Gets Fat.

Weight gain is not socially selective. "If your friends jumped off a cliff, would you jump too?" (If I had a nickel for every time my mom asked me that, every store I went into, the employees would say, "Great, here comes the guy that pays with all nickels.") Each individual has unique chemistry that is likely different from every other person in the world—much like a fingerprint. But if we look at the chemistry of an individual, we can begin to get an idea of what issues may be causing weight gain in that individual. That would explain how two friends could literally eat identical foods, yet one friend would gain no weight while the other friend is thinking about buying stock in Spanx.

One person has a body chemistry or functionality that is predisposed to create an environment where fat storage increases readily, while the other friend's body is operating in a manner that prevents that from happening. In my opinion, this is not a curse that you are just stuck with.

Your Fat May Be Saving Your Life

I don't mean that your fat may be saving your life if it helps you bounce off of oncoming traffic. It is more scientific than that. This topic will be an extension of the *I Love Lucy* example I made in chapter one under *How Medications Work*. As I said, when the liver is overwhelmed and can't remove enough toxicity from the body, the body can store junk in fat cells. This is sort of an emergency back-up plan to take a substance that is harmful and could wreak havoc on the body, and make that substance inert by shoving the toxic stuff into a fat cell. If it is stored in a fat cell, it won't pose any immediate threat. If the body didn't store this junk in fat cells, these toxins could upset the delicate balance of the bloodstream and we could literally die. In that regard, thank you, fat. Thank you for helping me avoid death today.

This is a major source of weight gain for a big percentage of the population. When looking at toxic substances that may need to be stored in fat cells within the body, medication is only one of the possibilities. The list of substances that may be considered toxic to the body could go on for the rest of this book. Things like pollutants in our air and water, chemicals in our cleaning products, and additives, pesticides and hormones that are found in our food. Even organic, natural foods that would normally be considered healthy can become toxic in the body as they rot and ferment, if not properly digested. What about the alcohol we drink, or cigarettes we smoke, or second-hand smoke we walk by? What about the plastics that seep from the bottle into the water we drink? How about the soda we pour into our faces, or the artificial sweeteners we ingest while we're trying to eat "low-fat?" Are you forgetting about the chemicals we make in our bodies while we're stressed or even just irritated because we can't believe that Jerry Springer is still on the air? Our bodies are well equipped to handle trouble from nearly every angle, but sometimes all the trouble combined is just too much. When the load is more than the body can handle, hello back-fat. This doesn't mean that every toxin has the ability to be stored as fat. However, anything that is adding to the toxic load still has the ability to trigger the body to store more junk in fat cells.

Obesity & Starvation

I believe that starvation is one of the leading causes of obesity, especially extreme obesity. When I say this to a crowd I always get looks that say, "We paid money to see this guy?" You may say to me, "Look, the guy is standing right there, he's four hundred pounds, he has a bucket of fried chicken in his hand right now... he's clearly not starving."

What I mean is this: He may be eating, but his body is not receiving the nutrition it needs. Chapter three explains the ins and outs of digestion, and for most readers it will be the most important chapter in this book. Here's the teaser: If a guy can break down and assimilate only ten percent of the nutrients in the food he is eating, doesn't it make sense that he would need to eat ten times as much food in order to get the nutrients required for his body to function?

Have you ever found yourself looking at people who are extremely overweight and thinking, "Why don't they do something about that? Don't they have any dignity?" You are allowing your ignorance of the subject to judge someone inappropriately. If you're a fat kid that gets teased day and night about your weight, know this: Someone finally has your back. Obesity is not about a lack of willpower or an individual who has no self respect. Obesity is about science and malfunctions in the body that are creating the excess weight.

While filming the documentary, *Why Am I So Fat?*, I talked to some of the most well respected celebrity trainers and nutritionists on the planet. Some of *them* don't even understand the truth behind weight loss, so of course the public view on the topic is going to be skewed. A few "experts" told me that if people just make a decision, they can change their habits. Sorry guys, there can be more to it than that. By the time you finish this book, and you understand the issues that can create obesity, you will know that no amount of willpower can overcome a body that knows how to get what it needs to survive and function. If you are obese, you will understand that it's not your fault and you will understand the steps you need to take to turn things around. You can also rest assured that, while you're doing the work to give yourself a new life, I'll be doing the work to explain the truth about obesity to every idiot that ever doubted you. Ready... BREAK!

Eat Real Food

This heading may sound like I'm speaking a foreign language to some of you. When I say real food, I mean food that grew out of the ground or fell off of a tree that grew out of the ground or came from an animal that peed on the tree while it was standing on the ground. That food doesn't include ingredients that were created in a laboratory. It's just food. Vegetables, eggs, animal proteins, fruits. These are real foods. These are the things that your body recognizes as real food. Do you really think your body recognizes squirt cheese as real food?

I know a package out of the vending machine is convenient and it's cheap. But you're going to pay for it one way or the other. You can either spend your money on real food, or you can start sending your local hospital a check every month, because sooner or later, that is where your money is going to end up. This doesn't mean that you can never eat anything processed. Our bodies are designed to remove junk safely when the body is not overwhelmed. What I am saying is this: Every meal you eat that is made of real food is giving your body nutrients it can actually use (as long as you digest it). Every meal you eat that is made from processed, chemical-ridden ingredients that you can't spell, is giving your body a problem it has to deal with. Be nice to your body now and it may let you poop your pants less when you're older.

I go over real food more in chapters thirteen through fifteen. For now, just know that adding in real food as often as possible can be a huge step in the right direction.

Shut Up About The Calories Already

Yes, I understand that I'm about to rock your whole belief system. I understand that you've purchased fourteen calorie counting books, you have a poster that hangs on your kitchen wall listing the calorie content of every food on the planet, and you just downloaded a new app called *Calorie Genie*. (I apologize if there really is a *Calorie Genie* and I just made fun of you. I honestly just made that up. But if that is your product and it's real, please consider getting a better name.)

"But nearly every diet I have ever followed had me count my calories. Every nutritional expert in our government has told me to burn more calories than I eat." Yes, I know. There is a reason you're not using those diets anymore, and that most of those government officials are big fat guys. Counting your calories is about as effective as painting your car with Crayons. It's very time consuming, you don't get the result you were hoping for, and the little sharpener always falls out of the back of the box... Maybe that last part only happens with the Crayons scenario. But counting calories still stinks.

Do you even know how they determine calories? Scientists burn the food in a bomb calorimeter, which is a box (or in some cases, a big fancy oven looking device) with two chambers, one inside the other. The researchers weigh a sample of the food, put the sample on a dish, and put the dish into the inner chamber of the calorimeter. They burn the food within the inside chamber, and then measure the rise in temperature of water kept in the outside chamber. Each degree the water temperature rises equates to one calorie, generally speaking. Tell me this, where in the human body is there a high temperature oven? Or even a flame if we're comparing to those calorimeters that burn food using a flame. There's not. Some people are very flamboyant, but even these folks don't have an actual flame. This method is so far from human physiology, it's a joke.

Calorie experts tell us that a calorie is a calorie is a calorie. They tell us that the unit of energy measured by a calorie in broccoli is the same as a calorie found in banana cream pie. Yes, that is true when looking at a petri dish found in a lab. The problem is, humans are not a petri dish and we all process those calories differently. Therefore, it's not about the calories that you consume. It's about your body's ability to turn those calories into fuel. If your body has a problem processing carbohydrates, or fats, or properly digesting protein, those foods are not converted to energy according to the number of calories they contain. If we all processed foods the same way, this calories in calories out formula would be a beautiful thing. Unfortunately, we all process food differently and this calorie counting method is just one more idea that confuses and frustrates those who can't lose weight.

The real benefit to counting calories, and why some people succeed when they start cranking out the math, is simply that this calorie counting process makes you conscious of what you're eating. It lets you see exactly what you are shoving down your gullet. That's more valuable than just about anything else you can do. When I bring on new obese clients, I tell them that I won't even train them unless they're willing to journal everything they eat. Getting a true visual of what you consume in a day is an amazing tool.

Calories are okay to sort of get an idea of what you're eating, but the whole system is actually fictional. Treating the measurement of your food like you require the accuracy of a NASA mission is a waste of time and effort. If you don't believe me, try eating 2200 calories per day of just chicken, eggs and green vegetables for two weeks. For the following two weeks, try eating 2200 calories per day of Twix bars and let me know which two week period you had better weight loss results.

What you eat is much more important than the total number of calories. I know that you have heard over and over again that if you burn more calories than you eat, you will lose weight. That didn't work out, did it? You can use calories for a benchmark, but what you're eating is far more important. I don't have any of my clients count calories at all.

It's more important to get your digestion working properly and implement eating real food that the body can process than to know the precise caloric identity of a food. A 100-calorie piece of processed snack food will almost always create more fat storage than 200 calories of real food that is optimal for your specific chemistry. (Please don't turn this ratio into some type of modified calorie counting rule.)

Later in this book I talk about the benefits of coconut oil with weight loss, how to use it, who qualifies to use it, etc. But to make my point about calories, coconut oil has 120 calories per tablespoon. It also has fourteen grams of fat (thirteen grams of saturated fat). I consume four to six tablespoons of coconut oil every day. Basically five hundred calories before I even add in any of my meals and I still eat four to six meals every day. Meaning, for many calorie counters, I consume a third of your daily calorie intake in just coconut oil. (Note: These high levels of fat and extra calories don't scare my six-pack away like many would believe.) Most of my clients who qualify to use coconut oil consume similar amounts to aid in weight loss.

It's not about the calories. It's about the choices. This topic will make even more sense when I cover how to avoid becoming a crazy person while you're losing weight. But, if the calorie game is so deeply burned into your brain that you're having a hard time moving past this right now, just know that one of us is right. Either I'm right and there is hope for you, or all those calorie counting idiots are right and you are destined to be overweight. I can't wait to find out which one it is. I'm rooting for my team because I don't think anyone is destined to be overweight if that person has the proper knowledge and is willing to turn that knowledge into understanding and implementation.

"Your body keeps an accurate journal regardless of what you write down."

-Unknown

Fat Is The Symptom, Not The Cause

There are countless conditions that are now associated with being overweight: Hypertension, Type II Diabetes, high cholesterol, etc. It seems like every doctor will tell you that if you just lose weight, many of those conditions may improve. Countless studies have shown that if you lose just X% of body weight, you can greatly increase the chance of improving Type II Diabetes, or high blood pressure, etc. But this is backward thinking, in my opinion. I'm not saying that my opinion matters the most, but in this book it does.

My view goes like this: The fat is not causing your hypertension. The fat has not given you Type II Diabetes. You don't need cholesterol medication because you are fat. The foods that you are eating, and the way your body is processing those foods, are the causes behind those issues. These are the same causes that are making you fat. If you understand what I'm saying, you can see that, yes, if you made the changes that allowed you to drop some weight, those changes could also improve any number of these conditions. But to view this scenario the way it is explained to us by the medical world will only confuse you, and may point you in the wrong direction.

If you understand that the direct cause of all these issues is either the choices that you're making or the way that your body is processing those choices, then you can do something about it. But, if you go along with what you hear in the media, from your doctor, or in pharmaceutical advertisements, and you believe that you have a "fat gene" or slow metabolism, or thick bones, you may feel like there's nothing you can do about it.

If you think your fat is causing the problem and you're genetically predisposed to own that fat forever, what choice do you have? You may as well have another slice of chocolate cake and enjoy what little time you have left, right? Are you starting to see why so many people feel like they have no other choice but to use medications, or have surgery, or other drastic measures? The outlook is hopeless out there. The good news is, the outlook is fiction. It's not true. It's entertaining and it sells products, but it's not true. Take the movie *The Avengers* for example. This was a work of fiction. It was funny, exciting, and very entertaining, but that stuff didn't really happen. It was all made up. Weird, huh?

The exciting part for you is that you do have choices. You have options, and this book gives you the tools you need to make those options work for you. It's going to take effort. Don't think it will be easy. But if you read through this book, your days of thinking that you are hopeless will be over. You may still choose to do nothing about your weight. Some people aren't interested in putting effort toward their goals. That's okay. Sometimes effort is not that fun. But you will know there are steps you can take to figure out what will work for you, and you will know those options will be here for you when the time is right.

I know I haven't gotten to any of those steps yet, but I'm just too excited. I have to ask... Do you think you're going to be ready to do the work? If you are, it is going to be so fun to hear from you once you begin your journey. Don't think I get tired of hearing success stories. It's the best part of my day so keep them coming. You know what? If you're a little gutsy, you should tweet to me right now at @kickitinthenuts. Say, "Hey Tony, I'm in chapter two and I'm ready to do the work." When you say something out loud, especially where others can see it, it makes the follow-through a whole lot easier. C'mon. Tweet it up.

"You may be born with a genetic map, but that does not mean you have to take the trip."
                                                                    -Me

Working With A Health Coach

Many topics in this book will be very simple, while some will get a little advanced. Keep in mind that there are professional health coaches around the world who understand how to look at your individual body chemistry and provide you with answers that you're looking for. In chapter sixteen I discuss how to find a professional near you. For now, if at any time you feel overwhelmed, know that help is available.

What To Expect

In this book, you're going to find answers. Answers to questions that you may have had your whole life. Most people who spend their life dealing with discomforts or issues feel like that's just the way it is for them and there's nothing they can do about it.

Issues like:

- Cravings
- Constipations
- Chronic Diarrhea
- PMS (if you're a menstrual-cycle-type person)
- Weight Gain
- Acid Reflux

The list goes on and on. Guess what? You can do something about it—all of it.

Wha'd He Say?

In this chapter, you learned:

- An individual may be storing fat for a combination of reasons, and these reasons can vary from person to person.
- Excess fat can be more than just "too much of the wrong foods." Body fat is a way the body can store toxins, like medications, chemicals from our food or environment, or even food that did not get properly digested.
- Fixing common digestive issues is a major priority when it comes to weight loss.
- You can count your calories or you can smash your hand with a brick. Both options are not very fun and rarely bring a long-term positive result.

CHAPTER THREE

Digestion

Everything Goes Back To Digestion

You will likely be surprised to learn that, in nearly every case of obesity, it all goes back to digestion in one way or another. If a lack of digestion is one of the most common underlying causes for issues that create obesity, don't you think it's possible that less severe digestive issues could also be contributing to the twenty pounds you'd like to get rid of? When I talk about digestion, I'm talking about people's ability to properly break down the foods they are eating. We all tend to assume that if food goes in one end and poop comes out the other, everything is working as planned. That is not always the case. Digestive issues are actually much more common than you might think. To illustrate: Line up 100 high school boys. You will likely find that the percentage of guys whose pants do not fit properly coincides with the percentage of people in this country who have some type of digestive issue. I know! That's a really high percentage. (And why don't they buy pants that fit... why?)

Diet is what a person eats but nutrition is what the cells see. Nutrition not making it to the cells is where we find the big disconnect. People think that if they focus on foods that are higher in specific nutrients, calcium for example, they're improving their calcium levels with these food choices. Little do they realize, if the body can't properly break down the food they are eating, they're just treating their toilets to calcium-rich poop.

That's what we're doing when we digest. We're breaking down that food into elemental parts that can be used by the body. Believe it or not, the body cannot run on a peanut butter sandwich any more than your car can run on crude oil. It just won't work. However, what the body *can* do is break down that peanut butter sandwich into minerals, amino acids, fats and sugars—and then use those nutrients. Your body needs those nutrients. When digestion is not working properly and you can no longer break down your food enough to pull the required nutrients out of what you have eaten, bodily systems can begin to fail, just like your car would fail if it ran out of gas.

In order for digestion to function properly, there are processes that MUST be in place for all the nutrients to be pulled from the food you eat. With digestive issues, not only are you missing out on nutrients, but undigested food now becomes a problem that your body has to deal with. If food is not digested, it rots and ferments, which creates gases and toxins. This explains how it doesn't really matter if you're eating organic, extra-virgin, all-natural, grass-fed, hormone-free lima beans washed by the prince of New Guinea. If you can't digest it, it will rot and ferment, creating garbage in your body.

Having reached this point of the book, you should have a basic understanding of how fat cells can be a tool for the body to store junk. Can you see how it might not matter what you eat if you can't digest it properly? Any food can result in excess stored fat if that food can't be broken down. This is the biggest piece of the puzzle that is missing from the weight loss industry. This is how I cheat. This is why I have clients who lose two hundred pounds in 9 ½ months. On top of amazing weight loss results, if these digestive issues exist for you, correcting them can improve a whole lot more than your waistline.

Remember, the methods I explain in this chapter are not magical weight loss secrets for everyone to implement. If you don't have any digestive issues, following the suggestions in this chapter won't do very much. First, figure out if you need help with your digestion. To give you a benchmark, out of twenty clients who come to me, only one of them will appear to have a properly functioning digestive system. Some readers won't need to follow all the guidelines in this chapter; but if you have weight to lose, odds are great that you could do something to improve your digestion.

When looking at an individual, I like to know as much about his or her chemistry as possible. Because this is not always an option, there are questions you can ask to get a good sense of how your body is operating. In chapter seven, I add self-tests you can run. Those, coupled with the following questions that you can ask yourself, will allow you to get a great picture of the exact nutritional changes that may benefit you the most.

How's Your Digestion?

In case you failed the last quiz miserably, I'll include a few of the same questions below to give you another chance to get a better score.

(1) Do you frequently pass gas?
    YES NO
(2) Do you often burp after meals or feel bloated? (Even just small burps.)
    YES NO
(3) Does your meal ever feel like it's sitting in your stomach like a rock for too long?
    YES NO
(4) Do you crave sweet or salty foods?
    YES NO
(5) Do some foods make you nauseous?
    YES NO
(6) Is your stool sometimes lighter than the color of corrugated cardboard?
    YES NO
(7) Do you ever experience heartburn or acid reflux?
    YES NO
(8) Have you recently taken any antacids or acid reflux medications?
    YES NO
(9) Are you frequently constipated?
    YES NO
(10) Do you frequently experience diarrhea or a loose stool?
    YES NO
(11) Do you ever see undigested food in your stool?
    YES NO
(12) Do you seem to gain weight no matter what you eat?
    YES NO

If you answered yes for one or more of those questions, you should pay special attention to this chapter.

If you answered yes for two or more of those questions, you will likely need to take action in order to get your digestion back on track.

If you answered yes for three or more of those questions, this chapter will likely change your life.

The Digestive Summary

Digestion is such an important factor when it comes to weight loss and a bevy of other health issues, that I've dedicated this entire chapter to explaining the whole system. I even explain strategies you can implement right away to begin to improve your digestion. That way, by the time you get to chapter seven and begin to figure out how whacked your chemistry is, at least you will have already taken steps to improve digestion and you'll be on your way to being a real human. Stand clear because you're going to enter biology class for just a few minutes. I promise to avoid any frog dissecting flashbacks.

When we eat, our stomachs make hydrochloric acid (HCL). This stomach acid, as it is often called, has a pH of around 0.8. The pH scale goes from zero to fourteen. Zero means acidity to the max. Fourteen means alkalinity to the max.

When contents of the stomach (what we eat and drink) are mixed with this stomach acid, that combination will ideally have a pH between 2.0 and 3.0, which is still very acidic. The acidic product created by mixing stomach acid with the food you eat then goes into the duodenum (first ten inches of the small intestine). The other half of the digestive process comes from the bile that is produced by your liver. (I say "half" loosely because there are other factors that contribute to digestion that are not important for this explanation. But for the most part, the main factors in digestion are the acid created in the stomach and the bile produced by the liver.) Between meals, bile is stored in the gallbladder where it is concentrated up to 18 times. When acid product from the stomach moves into the duodenum, bile from the gallbladder is dropped onto this acid product. In the same way that HCL is acidic, bile is alkaline (which is the opposite of acidic).

Bile meeting stomach acid is like dropping baking soda onto vinegar, just like at least one sixth grader does every year when he makes his version of a volcano for his science fair project. In fact, you should try that now. You don't need to build the whole volcano, but you can put a little bowl in your kitchen sink, put a couple teaspoons of baking soda in the bowl, and then slowly pour in a little vinegar. You'll hear a sizzle and see it start to foam up. C'mon, really do it! All the cool kids are doing it. It's a great visualization of what can happen when two substances with opposite pHs meet.

This is the magic of digestion. When the body drops bile onto the contents that comes from the stomach, you get a sizzle, and this is what you're living on. This is what makes everything that was in the food break apart and become available for your body to use. Without this sizzle, foods you eat can't be assimilated. Nutrients and minerals can't be properly extracted and utilized by your body if this action is missing. That's why you hear so many people say, "Health is like a science fair project." Okay, I've never heard anyone say that; but if you don't have that sizzle in your digestion, you might as well be that 12-year-old holding the volcano with an "F" on it because the lava didn't come out. You've got to have the sizzle.

If there isn't enough stomach acid, there won't be that sizzle. If there isn't enough bile to drop down onto the food that was mixed with the stomach acid, there won't be that sizzle. In order for digestion to work properly, every step of that process has to be active. Otherwise, instead of a sizzle, you get more of a fizzle; and you may break down just a very small portion of your food, or your food will partially break down by processes of rotting and fermenting. This rotting and fermenting creates chemical reactions and gases that can cause bloating, burping, nausea, bad breath, upset stomach, and all kinds of other non-fun stuff. Have you ever been around someone who had breath that smelled like a garbage can? Most people look at bad breath as a dental hygiene issue, and it can be; but more often than not it's a situation of, "I have food rotting in my stomach and intestines and the stench it creates is coming out of my mouth." Yes, I know you've met that guy.

This repulsive rotting of last night's dinner can also be the reason you don't feel like eating the next morning. Many of you who always skip breakfast truly have no appetite when you wake up. Some people are even nauseous because last night's dinner still hasn't fully digested.

Their bodies are telling them, "Look, I haven't finished dealing with this garbage you sent down here last night, please don't dump anything else on top of it." By improving digestion, your morning appetite can also improve.

Give Me Acid Or Give Me Death

A bit of a drama queen? Maybe. Maybe not. A lack of stomach acid can be a huge health concern that can result in even bigger health concerns. One of those being a boat-load of fat in your pants.

Here are a few of the issues that can come from a need for more stomach acid. I explain some of these further in chapter four when I cover elimination.

- Almost every nutritional deficiency stems from either a lack of stomach acid or a lack of bile flow. Poor food selection is usually the third factor.
- Burping or bloating. Bloating is almost always due to a lack of stomach acid.
- Frequent stomach discomfort after eating.
- Acid reflux or heartburn. Yes, reflux is usually caused by NOT ENOUGH acid, not too much acid like you see in advertisements. It's one of the biggest health mistakes being made by millions of people today.
- Chronic constipation. I mention another frequent cause in chapter eight; but a lack of stomach acid is often a factor, if not the main cause.
- The door is open for bad critters to sneak into your body. Stomach acid is the barrier that blocks harmful organisms from entering through the digestive tract.

Improving Your Stomach Acid

If you need to improve your stomach acid, there are supplements you can use to boost your body's ability to correct these functions. But, before I teach you how to use Betaine HCL supplements to recover your proper stomach acid function, I need to give you a huge WARNING. READ IT! DON'T IGNORE IT!!!!

*** HCL Warning ***

If you're going to use HCL, be sure to also use Beet Flow (explained below in *You Need Good Bile Flow*) or a similar product. I never allow any of my clients to use HCL unless they are also using Beet Flow. If you don't have your bile flowing correctly and you add more acid into the stomach, you could create a duodenal ulcer or diarrhea issues. I cover all of this in more detail in chapter four. I just want to make sure you understand not to use HCL without also using Beet Flow. It is also imperative to read *How to Use HCL Supplements* below before you begin supplementing with HCL.

Why Use HCL

We all know the body makes stomach acid. But when we hear about stomach acid, it's usually how people have "too much" acid and that's why they are dealing with heartburn or acid reflux issues. There is a lot of brilliant marketing by the pharmaceutical companies when it comes to stomach acid and why it might be a good idea to turn acid off, and I believe it the same way I believe that a mime is a talented artist. In Appendix A, I explain why people really get heartburn and reflux, but let's first look at why "turning off" your stomach acid with drugs is one of the worst possible things you can do for your long-term health.

Hydrochloric acid (HCL) is the protector of the human body. Let's say you are eating at the buffet and you're taking in viruses, bacteria, and microorganisms because you scoop up the salad the kids sneezed on a few minutes earlier. While you eat from this salad bar, you are taking in all this filth and you are eating undercooked hamburger and chicken drumettes that were dropped on the floor. The truth is you don't really know what you are getting. Keep in mind that I worked at a salad bar when I was a kid, and my only rule was that being funny in front of the cute waitresses was far more important to me than delivering clean, sanitary food to all the patrons that came in on coupon night. Your food doesn't even need to be dropped on the floor by a zit-faced high school kid to have bacteria or other little creatures on it. Even the food you clean and prepare at home can have some little ninja-like varmints that make it through the cleaning process. (Varmints! 500 points to me for fitting in a Yosemite Sam reference.)

That's where HCL becomes such a hero. Anything that comes into YOU (any microorganisms, bacteria, or other types of bad guys) is going to die in an acid bath. That stomach acid is the protector of the mechanism that is YOU. The hydrochloric acid function of the stomach is your knight in very disgusting armor. When you take a drug that turns that barrier off, you're opening the door to anybody that wants to come in and raid the pantry (you are the pantry in this scenario). That's why two people can eat the same meal and one will get food poisoning and have projectile fluids coming out of both ends, and the other person will just say, "The fish didn't taste right, did it? Oh, and sorry about your luck." One person had the proper level of stomach acid to kill whatever little bad guys were still living on that fish; and the other person is praying to the porcelain god, vowing to never eat seafood again.

The point is, you want that acid function to be in the stomach because it is the gatekeeper. It's the lock that keeps all the hoodlums out. I don't want you to think that taking medication for acid reflux or heartburn is the only reason a person may lose that acid function. There are many ways a person can produce less than the proper levels of acid. There are also many reasons the acid function may not fully recover for years, or even decades.

The body needs minerals in order to generate stomach acid. However, the body needs stomach acid in order to fully break down foods and pull minerals out of those foods. Without digestion, you can't assimilate minerals, but without minerals, you can't create proper digestion. See how someone could get stuck in a bad situation for a long time? Using HCL supplementation can allow you to manufacture proper digestion so you can pull the minerals out of the food you are eating. Once the body has enough minerals, the stomach can often begin to make an appropriate amount of HCL. At this point, the HCL supplementation can often be reduced until the body is making plenty of its own HCL— and then the supplementation can be removed altogether. Depending on your mineral reserves, food choices, and many other factors, this process can take weeks, months, or longer.

How to Use HCL Supplements

Hydrochloric Acid (HCL), also labeled as Betaine HCL, is the most widely needed digestive supplement in my opinion. It's also the one that comes with the most important instructions. This is NOT a supplement you want to take willy-nilly. (Isn't it amazing that such a ridiculous phrase like "willy-nilly" could become so widely accepted? That bugs me.) Here is a list of important guidelines to follow while using HCL supplements:

- HCL capsules should always be taken in the middle of the meal and chased by at least one bite of food. If the capsules were to get stuck in your esophagus and dissolve there, it could feel like heartburn.

- Start by taking one capsule with a meal containing no starches. This means avoid foods like potatoes, bread, pasta, cereal, rice, etc. If you don't feel a warming sensation in your stomach, or any other new digestive discomfort, about twenty minutes after the meal, you know it's okay to move up to two capsules at your next meal. You can continue in this manner until you reach a maximum of five capsules per meal.

- Most people will hold at five capsules per meal for months. However, if you begin to feel a warming sensation after your meal, you know you have taken too many capsules. At your next meal, you can reduce by one capsule and hold at that dose until you feel a warming sensation again. This is telling you that your body is starting to make more of its own HCL and you can begin to reduce the amount you are adding in.

- Be sure to adjust your dose according to the amount of protein in each meal. If you have a meal with very little protein, you may need to reduce the number of capsules you use with that meal.

- If you experience any diarrhea or loose stool issues after you begin to use HCL, reduce what you are taking until you can improve your bile flow using the suggestions found below in *Improving Your Bile Flow*. If you have more acid than your bile flow can handle, that can create a loose stool issue. This may not mean that you don't need the acid, you may just need to improve your bile flow before you can handle more acid. If you experience this issue, read more about loose stool issues in chapter four.

- Some people will never feel a warming sensation and that is okay. If you no longer feel bloated after meals and you are no longer having little burps, any reflux issues, or any digestive discomfort, you can try to reduce your dose at that time and see how you do. You may be able to eventually reduce to zero capsules and your body will continue making enough HCL on its own.

- If you experience magnified acid reflux when you begin using HCL, be sure to read about acid reflux in Appendix A so you know what steps to take to correct this.

You Need Good Bile Flow

This one issue alone may be the reason that so many diets you tried in the past failed. Bile is what allows us to emulsify the fats we eat so they can be used by the body. All food is either carbohydrate, protein or fat. To process the fats, you need bile. Bile is not only needed for proper digestion, bile is also the main exit pathway for filth and toxins from the body. I already talked about how junk that can't be removed can often get stored in fat cells, so this is a huge factor.

Here are a few of the issues that can come from a need for improved bile flow.

- Almost every nutritional deficiency stems from either a lack of stomach acid or a lack of bile flow. Poor food selection is usually the third factor.
- Passing gas. It can be a big indication that bile is not flowing correctly.
- Weight gain.
- Chronic diarrhea or issues like colitis, Crohn's, IBS, etc.
- Duodenal ulcer.
- Chronic acne.
- Stool color that is sometimes lighter than corrugated cardboard.

Improving Your Bile Flow

In chapter nine I talk about an imbalance that can cause your bile to become too thick and sticky and encumber its ability to flow correctly. For most people, however, using a supplement made predominantly of beet greens is enough to correct the problem. Beet greens have an amazing ability to help thin the bile so it will flow properly. Unfortunately, you would likely need to eat an entire bucket of beet tops on a daily basis in order to get the effect you're looking for. A concentrated supplement is far more effective and will allow you to avoid eating meals fit for a horse.

There are many beet supplements out there, but few contain as much of the beet green as Beet Flow from Empirical Labs. This is the one I use with my clients. It is absolutely the most expensive supplement I use, but it's well worth the money. If you are willing to do the work to correct digestion, this upgrade could help improve any number of ailments you are dealing with, reducing the number or remedies you may buy in an attempt to fix your woes. In this regard, investing in Beet Flow can turn out to actually save you money.

Why Use Beet Flow

If you're going to use HCL, you need to use Beet Flow as well. You really need to make sure your bile is flowing correctly if you're going to be adding more acid to your stomach. That acid needs to be neutralized by bile when it reaches the duodenum. If you want to digest your food correctly, you need both sides of digestion working properly.

Improving bile flow will greatly help your liver remove filth from the body—filth that could otherwise be stored as fat.

How to Use Beet Flow

Most people use only two or three capsules per meal. You can take them before or during your meal.

Note: If you are on birth control medication, be sure to read about it in Appendix A. It will freak you out. Birth control medication has the ability to close off the gallbladder tube so bile cannot flow properly.

Add Digestive Enzymes

Enzymes are another factor of the digestive process. All living foods are meant to contain enzymes that actually help you digest that food better. Yet, with today's despicable farming methods, even many raw foods do not contain the needed enzymes to correctly digest those foods. On top of that, any time food is processed or heated over 118 degrees (pretty much any time you cook food), the enzymes are killed and you will not get the full benefit from that food. In order to fully break down the food you eat, you can supplement enzymes with your food. As we age, the body's stockpile of usable enzymes diminishes. People over thirty should be supplementing enzymes with their food. If you don't supply your body with the enzymes it needs, your body steals enzymes intended for repair processes and turns them into digestive enzymes, leaving fewer repair-enzymes for their intended use.

With certain imbalances, TOO MANY enzymes can facilitate deterioration. So, you want to take just enough to help you digest your food. Many enzyme companies promote taking unlimited enzymes but that is not recommended with certain imbalances.

How to Use Digestive Enzymes

Most people see improvement by using only one or two capsules per meal.

Where To Get Supplements

The beginning of chapter sixteen covers the world that is consumer supplement sales. There is a reason you hear so much good and bad about supplement use. Supplements are good only if you use the right ones for the imbalances you are dealing with, and they are good only if you use high quality products that can be properly absorbed. With many supplements, the person using them can absorb only a very small percentage of what is in them.

I'm not saying that the supplements I recommend are the only good supplements out there. They have simply brought the best results, in my experience. Consumers miss out sometimes since most high quality companies sell only through practitioners. Empirical Labs is a company that sells most of their products only through qualified professionals. Having a wider variety of quality supplements available to you can be another perk of working with a professional health coach. However, some of Empirical Lab's products are available to consumers as well, since these particular supplements are considered to be safe for people to use, no matter what their chemistry is (so long as they use a little common sense). This is the brand I implement most frequently for my own use.

Most health food stores sell some form of HCL. I just don't like a lot of them because they contain pepsin and other ingredients that can bother people's stomachs when they start to use more than one capsule per meal. I try to use straight HCL. Also, the capsules I use are 515mg, so if you get something different, be sure to adjust your number of capsules accordingly. I use HCL from Empirical Labs, which can be found on www.NaturalReference.com. This is the only site approved to sell Empirical Lab's products to the public. Beet Flow and the digestive enzyme I prefer, Digesti-zyme, can also be found on this website.

I like the enzyme Digesti-zyme because it contains cofactors, like zinc, that the body can use to make its own HCL. In this regard, Digesti-zyme can reduce how long you may need to supplement HCL.

Supplements Review

www.NaturalReference.com
Brand: Empirical Labs

Betaine HCL (See the HCL warning under *Improving Your Stomach Acid* in this chapter.)
1-5 per meal (In the middle of the meal.)

Beet Flow
2-3 per meal

Digesti-zyme
1-2 per meal

In chapter sixteen I go over other supplements that can be used for other imbalances. With many of those supplements, I am not as picky about the brand I use with my clients. But when it comes to correcting digestion, I haven't seen anything else work as well as these three.

Wha'd He Say?

In this chapter, you learned:

- Nothing will improve your overall weight loss efforts like taking steps to improve your digestion.
- Both sides of digestion are equally important. You must have enough HCL production and you must have proper bile flow.
- Few people with digestive issues are able to truly improve digestion without the temporary aid of supplements.
- Most people will benefit from the use of digestive enzymes.
- You can order Beet Flow, HCL and digestive enzymes from www.NaturalReference.com.

CHAPTER FOUR

Elimination & Digestion Gone Wild

Let's Talk Poop

There are two types of people in this world. There are stargazers and there are stoolgazers, and the stoolgazers fare better. There is a lot that can be learned from poop—specifically, how our bodies are operating and, especially, how well digestion is working. Better understanding the signs of digestive trouble can guide your efforts toward improving many issues.

We all know that we poop to eliminate waste from the body. Many don't know, however, that stool often moves at its level of acidity. Stool can move too quickly and be too loose when it is too acidic. Not only does this burn the intestines, but also, if the stool is moving too quickly, the body doesn't get the opportunity to absorb as many nutrients as it should. In chapter six, I cover how a lack of usable nutrients can create issues with cravings. If stool is not acidic enough, it can move too slowly and even lead to constipation.

Diarrhea and Loose Stool Issues

Since you don't want nutrients screaming through your intestines without being absorbed, any loose stool or chronic diarrhea issues must be corrected in order to speed up your weight loss progress. In most cases, a chronic loose stool is the result of a lack of bile flow. Using Beet Flow to improve bile flow can correct that issue. If this is not enough, be sure to read chapter eight and learn about the Catabolic Imbalance that can hinder bile flow and may need to be corrected.

When you get your Beet Flow and have been using it for a day or two, you can do what is called a Beet Flow Flush. I just take four Beet Flow capsules every thirty minutes for two hours (a total of four doses). This is just a one-time event and not the protocol I use daily. This can give your bile flow a quick boost and many will see improvement faster by using this technique when they start.

It's best to get a loose stool under control before you start to add any HCL supplementation. If you haven't, you could create a duodenal ulcer by constantly pushing more acid into the duodenum without the proper level of bile dropping in to neutralize that acid.

If you are dealing with Crohn's, colitis, or IBS, be sure to read about these topics in Appendix A.

Constipation

Though stool that is too loose can often lead to extreme cravings due to a lack of nutrient assimilation, constipation can lead to weight gain in a more direct manner. If a lack of stomach acid results in stool that is too alkaline and moving too slowly, that waste that was supposed to be removed out the back door (your butt) can get held up in the system too long. If waste is not removed properly, it can be re-absorbed through the intestinal walls and will need to be filtered out all over again. If a liver is already overwhelmed, the body can end up storing that waste in fat cells.

Increasing your stomach acid by supplementing HCL can be a great first step toward improving constipation. If that doesn't speed up your stool and relieve your constipation, be sure to read chapter eight. There I explain an imbalance called an Anabolic Imbalance that is commonly responsible for chronic constipation issues.

Don't ignore this problem. Your weight loss results will be greatly hampered, if not totally shut down, any time you are not having at least one good bowel movement per day.

Burping, Bloating And Passing Gas

To figure out if you're really bloating, here's the ultimate question. (This question works only for women because men are way too oblivious of their bodies to get this one.) Are your clothes tighter in the evening when you take them off than in the morning when you put them on? If you so much as have to think about it, you're probably not bloating, because a woman knows. She will say, "Yeah, they are tighter when I take them off." She knows, and if they are tighter, she is bloating. If the acid product in the stomach is not sufficient then people are going to grow bacteria in their tummies. When they grow bacteria in their tummies, they are going to produce gas. It is the same as making beer or wine or champagne or root beer; all of these things are fermented. When you ferment, you are going to get gas and the gas is going to bloat. Some people may feel very bloated, while others may experience more burping.

When I say burping, I don't mean these huge belches. I'm talking about those little burps that are hardly even noticed. Those little burps are usually a good sign that the stomach is not acidic enough. I see a lot of people who don't even realize that they're burping after their meals. Once I ask them, they come back later and say, "Hey, ya know what, I am burping after my meals and I never even noticed." Now, it's your turn to pay attention and see if you're burping too. You may be burping because of the gas created by undigested food rotting and fermenting, or because of the gases created by bacteria that are living in your stomach, or because of a combination of both. Taking stock of what is going on with your body is the first step to making improvements.

People think, "Everyone passes gas, what's the big deal?" The problem is most adults don't have their digestion working correctly anymore and that is why gas is so common. If you're passing gas, it's usually because your bile isn't flowing well enough. If your bile isn't dropping into the duodenum to meet the acid product from the stomach, you're not digesting properly.

Helping Your Liver

I include some thoughts about liver function in this elimination chapter because proper bile flow is such a vital part of how effectively your liver is taking care of business. I say this a lot, and I'll probably say it three or four more times in this book: In my opinion, the two most important factors for good health are digestion and liver function. I'm not trying to say that if people have a horrific imbalance in need of attention, or an extra limb growing out of the side of their head, that they first need to correct liver function. I'm just speaking generally when I say that the liver's ability to handle its affairs is a super big deal, especially when it comes to weight loss.

I've covered a multitude of factors that can reduce a liver's performance: Almost any medication, a lack of bile flow, bringing in more junk than the liver can remove, etc. Any of these things can trouble a liver; and if the liver isn't working optimally, eventually your body won't be working optimally either. Think of your liver like a huge ventilation fan that can clear smoke out of a kitchen or entire house. Growing up as a kid, my family lived in a big yellow two-story house. In the living room, just outside of the bathroom, was a huge ventilation fan that was built into the ceiling. It had a metal shutter-like covering that would open when the fan was on and then close when you turned off the fan. This prevented all the freaky, Floridian bugs from flying into the house when the gusting wind wasn't cranking from the fan blades.

My Mom had a friend who would come over to the house and smoke in the living room. Even at twelve years old, I hated cigarette smoke and didn't want to smell it in my house any more than I wanted to miss an episode of *The Muppet Show*. Whenever my Mom's friend, Margaret, was over for a visit, I would turn on this huge fan and immediately it would suck all the smoke out of the house, as if it never existed. It's not that the house wasn't big enough to hold Margaret and myself at the same time, it was just too disgusting when that fan wasn't on.

This is similar to how your liver works. To say that your body can't handle a few toxins coming in is far from true. The liver is your body's massive ventilation fan. As junk comes in, the liver moves it out to keep the system clean and operating smoothly. I came home from school one day in a thunderstorm to find that our electricity was out. There was Margaret sitting on the couch. I could barely make out her beady little eyes through all the smoke, but I knew it was her. I immediately turned around to leave the house and my Mom asked where I was going. "Out to get struck by lightning," I said. I guess I was obnoxious when I was a kid too. In the same way I was too miserable to exist in that house without the fan, you might be too miserable in your life without your liver working properly.

After all the medical doctors had their way with me, and my liver was trashed from all the drugs I was taking, it was tough to even walk by some substances, much less take them into my body. When the liver is overwhelmed and can't handle the current load that it's already dealing with, it can be arduous for people to find foods they can eat without feeling miserable. There were only three or four very clean foods I could eat without feeling horrible because my body couldn't deal with the chemicals and preservatives found in most foods. Now that I have improved my liver function, those things don't bother me because my body can handle the trouble and my liver can remove those substances.

When it comes to weight loss efforts, your liver can be your best friend if you help it function correctly. By improving bile flow and helping your liver remove more junk, you not only keep the body from needing to store junk in fat cells, you also allow the body to go into fat cells to remove junk that may have been stored for quite some time.

BIG NOTE: If you have had your gallbladder removed, that can be a problem. Good bile flow is required for proper liver function, and a gallbladder is required for good bile flow. If you've had your gallbladder yanked, be sure to read about gallbladder removal in Appendix A.

Conquering Our Food - Food Allergies & Sensitivities

When you eat a salami sandwich (and no, I'm not recommending that you eat a salami sandwich... it's just fun to say salami sandwich), the goal is to conquer that sandwich instead of having it cause all kinds of trouble and carry you off captive. Food allergies are a very hot topic these days; and people come to me all the time and tell me about the testing they had done for food allergies. They tell me their tests showed they're allergic to nuts, dairy, wheat, gluten, soy, pork, turkey jerky, the board game Parcheesi, and Lou Diamond Phillips. Well, at what point does this person have to leave Earth in order to eat lunch? He's been told that he's allergic to just about everything on the planet. If you get to the point where you can eat only things that resemble Al Roker, it might be time to understand food allergies.

You may have already come across some of the rules or diets to help those with food sensitivities. There are gluten-free diets, blood-type diets, food-combining diets, raw-food diets—this list could keep going all the way down to the "*Saved by the Bell*, Zack & Kelly" diet. Most of these diets can actually benefit some individuals, but many people who need to employ a diet like this in order to feel better could find similar relief by correcting any digestive issues. Once you can fully digest what you're eating, the need to complete the "Screech-free" phase of the Zack & Kelly diet becomes obsolete.

So, what are all of these theories about food based on? There are so many books and diets and "gurus" out there it's enough to make you lose your appetite, even if you did know what you were supposed to eat. So, who's right? Do I eat for my blood type? Do I alkalize? Do I avoid carbs? Do I eat whatever I want as long as it starts with the letter "B"? Who's right? Well, I don't know. Whose research was everybody using as a basis for fact when they came up with these diets? Maybe most of the test subjects they used did, indeed, thrive on the ice cream sandwich diet. But, if you're interested in how the human body works, which I know I am, you first need to know how that particular human's digestion is functioning. If digestion is not so great, there is no diet that will fix all that person's woes.

Improper digestion is the reason juicing and blending have become so popular. Many fancy-pants gurus advocate buying these blenders that cost as much as a car and can liquefy your iPhone in thirty seconds. They tell us that we need to liquefy our food or we can't pull the nutrients out. And they're right, if you're a person with horrible digestion. That's why so many people feel better when they start to juice—they're actually getting some nutrients into the system. I do find that these juicing maniacs get a little upset when they learn that simply fixing their digestion can give them the same benefit. "You mean it was unnecessary for me to blend my turkey meatloaf and brussels sprouts and drink it through a straw?"

Let me get back to the point and break down these food allergies a little bit. Enzymes can play a factor in food sensitivities. If people don't have the correct enzymes to break down a specific type of food, that food can give them trouble. Take dairy for example. Many cases of lactose intolerance are just situations where people are lacking the enzyme lactase. If they supplement this enzyme, they may see improvement with their intolerance. The Digesti-zyme supplement I mentioned in chapter three is a broad-based enzyme that includes lactase.

The main cause for food allergies, however, normally has more to do with improper digestion than a lack of enzymes. In chapter three, I talked about how your body can't use a peanut butter sandwich until that sandwich has been broken down into elemental nutrients. This same understanding is used when looking at food allergies. Once you break down that peanut butter sandwich, it's no longer a peanut butter sandwich. Instead, it is now minerals, fats, amino acids—the things your body needs and recognizes as nutrients that can be used to rebuild your body.

However, if you never break down that peanut butter sandwich because your digestion is not working properly, that food still has its own identity since it was never conquered. That identity says, "Hi, I'm a peanut butter sandwich." Well, there is no use for a "peanut butter sandwich" in the body. The body can use only the nutrients that are pulled out of that peanut butter sandwich once it has been broken down by a functioning digestive system. If this peanut butter sandwich enters the system absorbed by the bloodstream etc. and still has its own identity, it is looked upon by the body as an invader and will be attacked and removed. A peanut butter sandwich is not going to be recognized as something that can be used. For this reason, the defense system is going to run and scream and sound the alarms. As your immune system creates antibodies to deal with this invader, an imprint of those antibodies is saved in the "security files." Now, the next time you eat a peanut butter sandwich, all heck breaks loose as the system comes down hard on this "invader" and you can feel an "allergic response." And why wouldn't you? Your body just went to war against a peanut butter sandwich for cryin' out loud. You're not supposed to be trying to digest a peanut butter sandwich in your bloodstream using your immune system. **PLEASE NOTE: This is not to say that someone with a peanut allergy or something as severe and life-threatening as that should not take it seriously.** They absolutely should. That is not what I'm talking about here. Most of those individuals were born with an allergy like that. I'm talking about sensitivities that people have developed in their life due to an inability to digest, or conquer, their food.

Acid Reflux, GERD, & Heartburn

Acid reflux, GERD, and heartburn are all issues that normally arise from digestive issues. If you deal with any of these problems, be sure to read about them in Appendix A now. I promise chapter five will still be there waiting when you come back.

Wha'd He Say?

In this chapter, you learned:

- Become a stoolgazer to gain valuable information about how your digestion is functioning.
- Chronic diarrhea-type issues are often caused by a lack of bile flow. Since the acid product from the stomach was not neutralized by enough alkaline bile, the body marches the acid out the back door in a big hurry so you don't burn your intestines.
- Increasing bile flow can help your liver clean out more junk, so the junk doesn't get stored in fat cells.

CHAPTER FIVE

Keeping Insulin Levels Low

High Insulin Levels

Cravings are the reason that most of us eat too many starches, carbs or sugars. To simplify this chapter, I will just say "carbs" when I am referring to starches, carbs or sugars. However, when I say this, I am referring to foods that are higher in carbs. Many green vegetables contain carbs in small amounts, and that is great. When talking about the ability for carbs to spike insulin levels, I'm talking about higher-carb foods. Foods like bread, pasta, rice, cereal, baked goods, potatoes, fruit, desserts, etc. Carbs are converted to glucose (or sugar) in the body and foods higher in carbs, convert to higher levels of glucose. In any case, the fact that you are consuming these carbs isn't even the major problem. The real villain in most people's weight loss story is how eating these carbs can push insulin levels too high, too often. Anytime we eat carbs, our insulin levels spike in order to sweep the excess glucose out of the bloodstream and into the cells. The more carbs taken in, the higher the insulin spike. Liquid carbs or sugars like juice, soft drinks, and alcohol spike insulin even higher because liquid hits the bloodstream faster.

Glucose levels can come down pretty quickly, but the insulin levels stay high a lot longer. The problem is, as long as your insulin levels are high, your body's ability to burn stored fat is impeded. There are more hormones involved in this total process, but viewing high insulin levels as the trigger that makes it all go bad is a simple way to explain it. High insulin levels also send the signal to your body to store fat. It says, "We have plenty of glucose to use here so store other fuel as fat in case we don't have glucose later." Make sense? So, the sugars are burned in a couple hours, yet your body can't access stored fat for fuel while the insulin levels are still high. No glucose and no access to stored fat means you don't have a good fuel source. Now, you start to crave more carbs because your body needs fuel to function. Even though the insulin isn't going to come down for another two or three hours, you eat a snack that's filled with carbs and your insulin spikes again, never giving the insulin a chance to come down and allow your body to burn fat for fuel. This pattern can result in insulin spike after insulin spike, all day long. Considering the way some people eat, do you see how it can be literally impossible to burn stored fat?

Charts & Food Examples

Let's look at examples of how certain meals could affect insulin levels and, therefore, fat storage. In the meal graphs below, I use a general scale from one to ten. I'm not using actual blood glucose or insulin numbers. This is a visual to show how high each level is on a scale of one to ten.

Meal 1 - 8:00 AM (Carb Count: 73 grams)
Bowl of oatmeal, whole wheat english muffin with jam, and a glass of orange juice.

If Phyllis eats meal 1 at 8:00 AM, in the graph below, we see her glucose (the dotted line) rise to a level 8 and her insulin (the solid line) follow right behind it. The shaded zone that tops out around 2.5 is the fat burning zone. Insulin levels need to be within this zone in order for your body to access stored fat and burn it as fuel. While insulin levels are outside that zone, not only can your body not access stored fat, but also your body will likely be storing *more* fat.

Meal 1 Graph

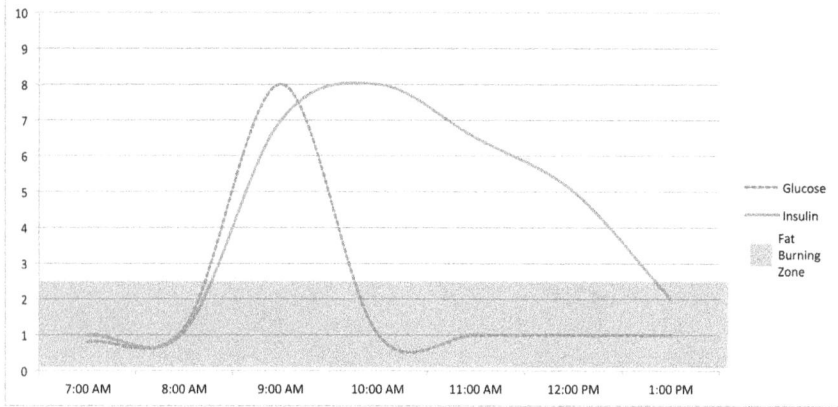

By 9:30 AM Phyllis' glucose has come down, but her insulin is still very high and will likely take a couple more hours to come down.

With glucose levels as low as they appear near 10:00 AM, the body would normally dig into fat storage and burn this fat as a fuel source. Yet, in the graph above, you can see that the high insulin levels block the body's ability to access stored fat, leaving Phyllis with no fuel.

What does Phyllis do? She eats a banana and drinks pomegranate juice because her friend saw an infomercial that stated pomegranate juice has health benefits.

Meal 2 - 10:00 AM (Carb Count: 59 grams)
Banana and a glass of pomegranate juice.

In the Meal 1 Graph you can see how insulin levels would have come down gradually, putting Phyllis back into the fat burning zone later that day. However, in the Meal 2 Graph below you can see that once she consumed Meal 2 with all those carbs (especially liquid sugars, which can spike insulin even higher than sugars in solid form) her glucose soars straight up again and another increase in insulin follows immediately. The sugar supplies her with an energy boost, but her insulin levels never have the chance to come back down before the sugars create another jump in insulin.

Meal 2 Graph

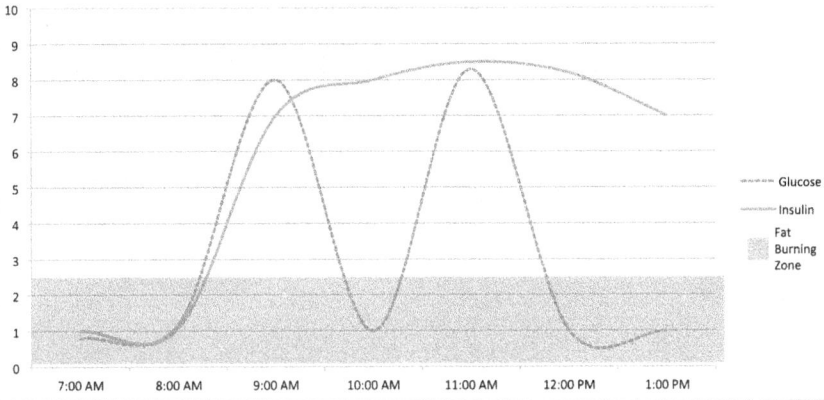

Meal 3 - 2:00 PM (Carb Count: 130 grams)
Turkey sandwich on whole grain bread with lettuce, tomato and fat-free dressing, side of brown rice and a fat-free mocha latte.

You can see that Phyllis was trying to "eat right" by selecting choices many consumers believe will lead to weight loss; yet, look at how this meal cranks her insulin levels off the charts in the Meal 3 Graph.

Meal 3 Graph

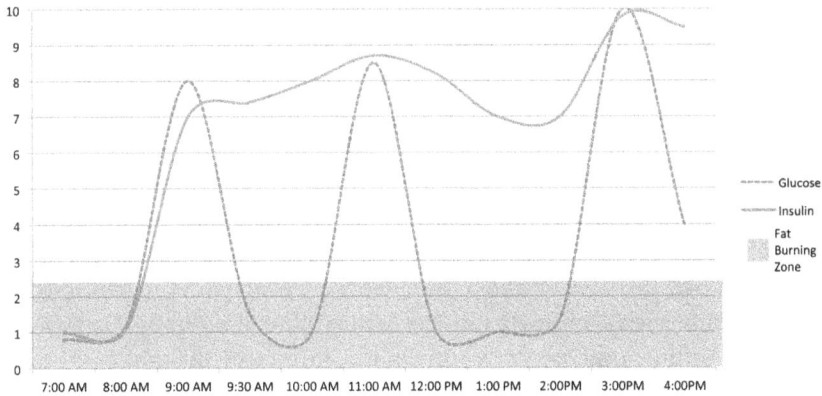

Meal 4 - 8:00 PM (Carb Count: 47 grams)
Small salad with ranch dressing and two rice cakes.

Phyllis tries not to eat too many calories late at night so she made a low-calorie meal. Too bad these low-calorie options still have high carbs. Rice cakes are one of the most nutrient-depleted, insulin-spiking foods you can eat, and many ranch dressings have more sugar than a candy bar. Graph 4 represents her glucose and insulin reaction to this meal.

Meal 4 Graph

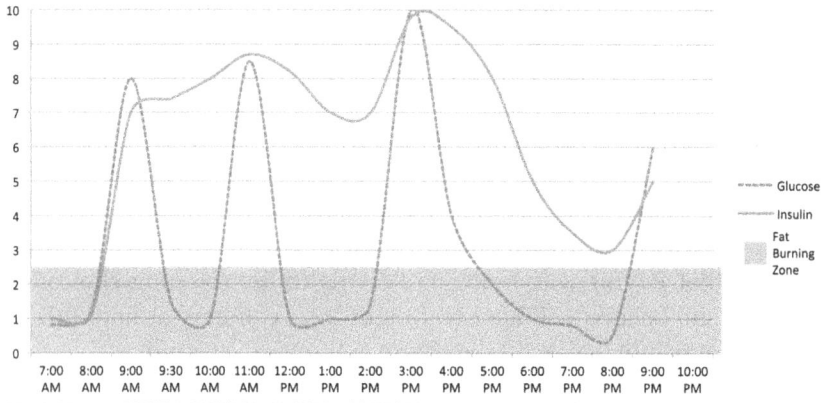

Oops - 8:20 PM (Carb Count: 64 grams)
One pint of Chubby Hubby ice cream.

An even bigger problem shows up after Phyllis eats her nighttime meal fit for a bird. Since she went six hours without eating, she is now ravenous. She already lost her mind and snapped at an elderly lady in traffic earlier that afternoon. "If your hair is that blue, you're too old to be driving!" I believe were Phyllis's exact words. Now, after her tiny dinner, she thinks she'll just have a few bites of ice cream. Ten minutes later she realizes she has wiped out the whole pint of Chubby Hubby. (By the way, if the food you're eating has Chubby in the name, you might want to pick another food.)

Oops Graph

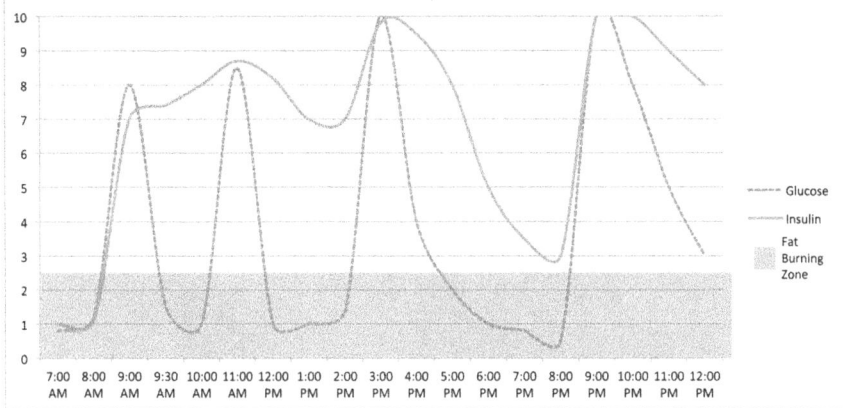

Looking at Phyllis' insulin levels over the span of the day, it's easy to see that, not only was her body unable to access stored fat for most of the day, she will likely stay out of fat burning mode for most of the night as well.

What would her insulin levels looked like with different choices?

Meal 1 Alternative - 7:00 AM (Carb Count: 2 grams)
Spinach omelet with butter, two turkey sausage links, and one cup of chamomile tea.

This meal provides a very nominal rise in insulin levels. Now, Phyllis can go right back into fat burning mode before it's time for a snack. She may be able to skip the snack altogether since her body will have the ability to access stored fat for fuel and she will have plenty of energy. But let's throw a snack in there anyway to see what happens.

Meal 2 Alternative - 10:00 AM (Carb Count: 18 grams)
Cottage cheese with berries.

This snack provides Phyllis with some needed carbs without spiking insulin levels too high.

Meal 3 Alternative - 1:00 PM (Carb Count: 3 grams)
Grilled chicken caesar salad without croutons.

The caesar dressing contains good fats to help keep Phyllis satiated.

Meal 4 Alternative - 4:00 PM (Carb Count: 6 grams)
Protein shake and a handful of raw almonds.

Meal 5 Alternative - 8:00 PM (Carb Count: 5 grams)
Lamb chops with sautéed broccolini and asparagus.

Alternative Meals Graph

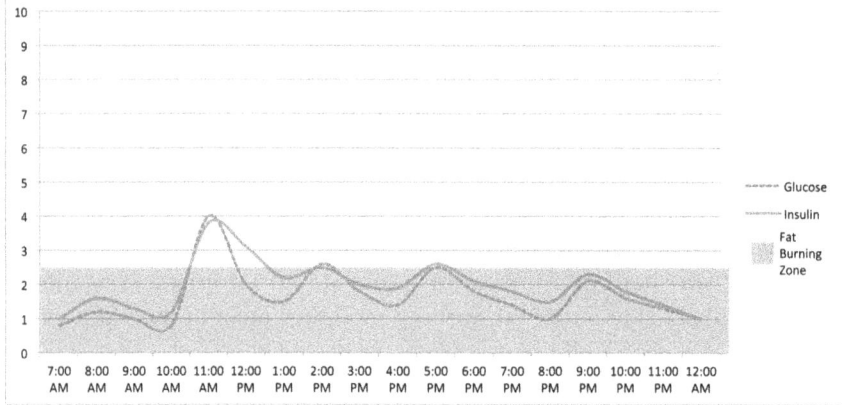

Though Phyllis had one small insulin spike mid-morning, look at the extended periods in the day where she is able to access stored fat and burn it for fuel.

When I teach you about cravings in chapter six, I show you how to reduce carbs without turning into a mental case. Then, and only then, will you be able to take complete control of your insulin levels. This is the science behind weight loss. There is no getting around this science. If insulin levels are high, you will not burn much stored fat, and in most cases you will end up storing more fat. The only difference from person to person is the strength at which the insulin operates, whether or not that person's cells are still receptive to insulin, and how much insulin needs to be utilized to move glucose into the cells.

This is one of the factors that allows some people to eat a high-carb diet with no weight gain. If their insulin is strong enough, they can move a large amount of glucose into the cells with a relatively low amount of insulin; therefore, they rarely have a big insulin spike. It's not the amount of sugar that we consume that necessarily dictates the amount of body fat we store. It's the level of insulin needed to move that glucose into the cells that dictates how long the body will stay in the fat-storage mode and out of the fat-burning mode. The more carbs consumed, the more insulin is normally needed to process those carbs; but the insulin is the driving force behind fat storage. If you can keep your insulin levels low, you can restrict the amount of fat your body stores and increase the amount of stored fat your body burns. That's it. It's called science.

Am I saying that everyone should go on a low-carb diet? No, I'm not. Many people don't qualify to go on a low-carb diet because they can't process other nutrients very well. If you take away their carbs, you will take away all of their fuel. They tend to get a little pissy when that happens. Therefore, if a guy wants to lose weight, but he doesn't qualify to reduce his carbs and lower insulin levels, the goal should be to correct those pathways that are restricting his ability to process other nutrients. Once he can use other nutrients, like fats and proteins, then he can work on reducing his carbs and bringing down his insulin levels.

3:00 PM Carb Cutoff

Keep in mind that some individuals will burn sugars better than fats and vice versa. In chapters seven and eight, I teach you how to look at your own chemistry to figure out what types of foods your body may be burning better than others. Let's also assume that you're already working on digestive issues you might be dealing with. That being said, the information below is all about trying to reduce the demand for high insulin levels for at least part of the day so the body can be freed up to better focus on other issues such as burning stored fat as fuel.

So, here's the trick... Try to eat any carbs before 3:00 PM on every day that you can get away with it. If you're done with carbs by 3:00 PM, that gives your body fifteen or sixteen hours that it can focus on burning fat, removing junk (that could otherwise get stored as fat) and taking care of all the tasks that make us healthy... all the jobs that the body is meant to do but often can't because it's being slammed with high insulin levels all day long. (Keep in mind that most foods have at least a small amount of carbs in them. Proteins and low-carb vegetables are a great choice in this scenario. You just want to avoid the carbs that will spike insulin levels.)

Many people like this trick because it allows them to have some of the foods that they like, just earlier in the day. In that way, you're not really depriving yourself of any one thing. That doesn't mean you should wake up and have two sandwiches, a bowl of pasta and whole box of cereal before 3:00 PM. You still have to eat healthy.

Then, once a week or so, when you want to go out with friends and eat a bit of carbs at night or have a drink, you don't have to be so concerned about it because you just had five or six nights in a row where you allowed your body to do what it needs to do. Maybe one week you have two nights that include more carbs and one week you have none. Even if you just eliminate most carbs after 3:00 PM three or four times a week, it's still better than having carbs every night—and you should still see some improvement. But please remember that any type of carbohydrate "bingeing episode" can rock a variety of systems in the body that can take up to seventy-two hours to recover from. So, while I am suggesting that you have fewer carbohydrates in the evening, overindulging in carbohydrates at any point during the day can really throw the body off its kilter. Some individuals will have more leeway while others may need to stick to this plan on a daily basis. It's just the knowledge of how the body works that will let you judge for yourself how often you want to implement this plan or not.

Those who have enough mineral in their systems to reduce carbs for the majority of their meals will be able to achieve much faster results. For those who need carbs because you don't have enough mineral in the system to function properly, this 3:00 PM carb cut-off plan can be a great way to still get results.

What Carbs Should I Eat?

In chapter seven, I show you how to figure out if the mineral levels in your system appear to be too low. Since you don't want to eliminate too many carbs if you have low mineral content, understanding which carbs are the best to eat can be helpful. The glycemic index explains the speed at which different carbohydrates convert to glucose and spike blood sugar levels. Searching for "glycemic index" on the Internet will bring up a variety of charts and tables showing the glycemic value of different foods. You might be surprised at some of the values you find. For example, potatoes have a glycemic value of 90 while white sugar is only 60. I'm not saying that white sugar should be a staple in your diet, but this shows that potatoes could have the ability to spike insulin levels more than sugar. If you are familiar with the glycemic index and want to continue using that form of carb measurement, I am okay with that. But I find another method a little more simplistic.

Active Carbs

I like to look at the "active carb" count of a food. Since fiber reduces how quickly the carbs in food hit your bloodstream, the higher the fiber and the lower the carbs, the better. To figure out the active carbs just subtract the fiber from the carbs and that will give you the active carbs. (In other words, the carbs that will spike your insulin.) If you can keep active carbs around 2g-20g for as many meals as possible, you'll be doing yourself a big favor in the realm of reducing insulin spikes.

For example, in the sample nutrition label image shown here, you can see the total carb count is circled and there is an arrow pointing to the fiber content. By subtracting the "Dietary Fiber" of 3g from the "Total Carbohydrates" of 13g, you have calculated that this particular food has an active carb count of 10g per serving.

Nutrition Facts
Servings Per Container 4

Amount per serving ½ cup

Calories 90	Calories from Fat 30
	% Daily value
Total Fat 3g	5%
Saturated Fat 0g	0%
Trans Fat 0g	0%
Cholesterol 0mg	0%
Sodium 300mg	13%
Total Carbohydrates 13g	4%
Dietary Fiber 3g	12%
Sugars 3g	12%
Protein 3g	4%
Vitamin A 80%	Vitamin C 60%
Calcium 4%	Iron 4%

The main thought to keep in mind is that, if you eliminate most carbs while your mineral content is low, you're going to have crazy cravings, end up bingeing like a madman, experience depression issues or, even worse, have a seizure. Your goal should be to include carbs that won't spike your blood sugar so high. Once you correct digestion issues and get more minerals in the system, you can reduce carbs further, if needed. You just don't want to drop your carbs too low in the beginning, while mineral levels are still too low. Including higher fiber carbs that have a lower active carb count, or are lower on the glycemic index, is a great way to hold off your cravings for things like chocolate, sweets, and complex carbs like bread, potatoes, rice or pasta.

Avoid Liquid Sugars

If fiber reduces the number of active carbs in a food, think of liquids as doing the opposite. Liquid sugars spike insulin levels faster and higher than most foods with a similar carb count. Liquids don't need to be digested or broken down, they just go right into the system. When you drink something like a soda, which can contain 39 grams of sugar, that liquid form of sugar could spike your insulin as high as three candy bars. Removing all forms of liquid sugar from your diet can improve your weight loss more than just about anything else you can do. Yes, even juice is a liquid sugar. Juice is just fruit without the brakes (a.k.a. fiber). Fruit was designed with those brakes for a reason.

The same goes for alcohol. Drinking "clear" alcohol does not make you immune to weight gain. It's still going to process like a liquid sugar and you're still going to pack on the pounds with every shot.

Intro To Cravings

The principles you learn in the next chapter about cravings will change the way you view weight loss. This really is the big kahuna. A big golden nugget was learning that it's high insulin levels that are causing you to store fat and restricting your body from burning stored fat. That's great. But that still leads you right back to trying to figure out how to limit carbs without waking up from a zombie-like state with a half-eaten bag of M&Ms in your hand. Understanding the need to reduce carbs is one thing; learning methods that will make that reduction easy for any carboholic... that will be your real pot of gold.

The good news is: You're still going to be able to have a variety of carbs if you want to; and many of you will be required to continue eating specific carbs because I don't want the insane asylums to be filled with nut-cases carrying my book around.

Your first job will be to follow the steps outlined in the next chapter to help reduce your cravings. I know you feel like saying goodbye to your pizza or your double fudge ice cream will be impossible, but I'm here to tell you it will be a piece of cake... except without the cake. When you start to give your body what it really needs, it will stop screaming for this junk all the time.

In chapter six, I teach you how you can find foods higher in carbs that won't spike insulin levels, and how to include medium-carb foods if your cravings are still hard to get past. The medium-carb foods will reduce any cravings and may slow weight loss a little, but should still allow you to continue seeing progress. And that is what you really want—progress.

Now, let's crack those cravings.

Wha'd He Say?

In this chapter, you learned:

- Consuming too many carbs can spike insulin levels. These high insulin levels block the body's ability to burn stored fat. High insulin can also send the signal to store more fuel as fat and may continue to do so for as long as those insulin levels are high.
- By consuming foods lower in carbs, you can keep your insulin levels down and allow your body to access stored fat and burn it as fuel.
- Some people do not qualify to remove too many carbs from their diet. If you have a low level of minerals in your system, you will need to consume more carbs.
- By eliminating carbs after 3:00 PM, you give your body an extended period of time for insulin levels to come down so the body can access stored fat and use it as fuel.

CHAPTER SIX

Cravings

How many times have you been excited to be doing so well on a diet, getting results and feeling good about yourself—only to have a craving come on that is so strong, you're certain it was beamed into your brain by aliens? You find a way to rationalize that eating these four cupcakes will somehow help you in your weight loss long term. You tell yourself that if I just allow myself to eat this one large pizza, I'll be perfect for the rest of the week. You may even tell yourself, "Yes, I understand the principles of the diet that I'm on, but obviously they didn't mean to leave out chocolate. How could I function without chocolate?"

Cravings destroy more diet efforts than any other single factor. If you never craved bad foods, any of the thirty diets you have probably tried may have worked for you. I talk about cravings throughout this book. Right now, I'll explain the issue that is usually responsible for cravings for most people; especially if you normally crave sugar, chocolate, carbs or salty foods.

Cravings can be a touchy subject for people and a tough issue they have dealt with for years, or even decades. Yes, there can be emotional baggage attached to cravings that goes all the way back to your first Easy-Bake Oven, or even earlier. But if you have emotional issues and are in need of finding a way past them, understanding what I'm about to explain to you can take the difficulty level of moving past them from a ten, all the way down to a one... if you're willing to do the work to correct this one circumstance. Here is how it works. If a person's salts (mineral content) are low, that person can have seizures. If a person's sugars are low, that person can have seizures. If salts and sugars are low at the same time, that person has an even greater chance of having a seizure. If your blood pressure is usually low, and you have other issues that can push your blood sugar very low too, that's the perfect recipe for some crazy, crazy cravings—the type of cravings where you might literally steal candy from a baby. (I'm sure you rationalized it by saying that the baby was very whiny and did not deserve the candy.)

When I discuss pH levels of urine and saliva in chapter seven, I explain the circumstances that can cause blood sugars to go too low. When a person's minerals and sugars go too low at the same time, this is the most common cause for cravings. This is usually why people crave salty foods, sweet and sugary foods, or carbs like bread, pizza or crackers (that can be converted to sugars). The body isn't so dumb. If salts are low, you can buffer them by raising your sugars and you'll be fine. The reverse is also true. If sugars are low, you can buffer them by raising your salts. The cravings are your body's way of helping you to raise either your salts or your sugars in order to keep you from pushing toward seizures.

Where most people think that something is wrong with them, or they just have no willpower, the truth is you can't compete with a body that knows how to get what it needs to continue functioning properly. Does that mean that these sugars or carbs are good for you? No; but don't you think your body would be more concerned with not having seizures than it would be with gaining weight? Doesn't it make sense that if the body recognized a "looming seizure" that would basically shut down the whole system, it would take steps to keep that from happening?

To get rid of cravings, people with low salts (or low blood pressure) can raise their mineral content by:

1. Using unrefined salt (like sea salt).
2. Using specific supplements.
3. Correcting any digestion problems that are keeping the body from properly breaking down food, so the mineral content can be assimilated by the body. If you're not digesting correctly, you're not getting the minerals out of your food.

I go over all those steps in detail after you are able to look at your specific body chemistry and figure out which of those steps, or what combination of those steps, are appropriate for you. Remember, this book is not about just doing things because they worked for someone else. This book is about figuring out what is right for you and your chemistry. If you have high blood pressure, I will include steps for you to take to tackle your cravings as well.

Just don't get ahead of me. I'm not saying that if you're craving sugar you're about to have a seizure. It just means the body is very defensive when it comes to having seizures, and it plans way ahead of time by sending out the signal for more things that can thicken the bloodstream and raise the minerals or the sugars. Your body doesn't know that you have cereal in the cupboard thirty feet away. It still operates under the assumption that you need to go out and hunt down a zebra or track down berries somewhere. Believe it or not, the body was not designed with "Special K" in mind.

The body may be feeling a little panicked about the low resources. The body may be sending a signal that you interpret as, "Hey... you... go to the store and get some double fudge ice cream and a box of those Nilla Wafers." This urge doesn't mean that a seizure is about to kick in. Even if you didn't eat anything else for another ten to twenty hours or more, you likely could still avoid a seizure.

If you've been struggling with your "relationship" with food for most of your life, you may have just received the biggest piece of information you will see in years. Again, a lack of minerals is not always the cause behind your cravings; it's just the most common. But the same goes for almost any craving. If you're having a craving, your body is looking for something that it needs, and your craving is merely your interpretation of that need. Your body could be needing fats or specific amino acids or vitamins. The possibilities are countless.

The important part is learning how to figure out what your body needs, and then don't be so stingy. Let your body have it. That doesn't mean if you're craving a rocky road sundae that you should let your body have it. It simply means there must be specific nutrients (or even junk that can be used in place of those nutrients) in that sundae that could help the body function better at that moment. Since simple sugars can be very easy for the body to break down and utilize, that can sometimes be what the body screams for in a pinch. Your body doesn't care that the sundae is going to spike insulin levels and make it so you can't button your pants anymore. Your body is just looking for anything it can use as a resource. Finding a way to provide your body with the nutrients that it truly needs will normally alleviate the craving for quick-fix junk, like sugar, that can come with its own set of problems. Much of this book will teach you how to do just that—how to give your body what it needs so your body will shut up and stop screaming, "Give me Sour Patch Kids!"

Correcting Cravings

If you know your blood pressure is low, I explain more steps you can take to correct cravings as you progress through the book. However, anyone with cravings can begin by adding healthy fats. Fats can be a big part of what your body is missing since so many people still live in the fictional world of the eighties that told us to reduce our fat intake. Since nutritional fats are required for so many functions, including brain function and cellular repair, cravings can be a big signal that you're not getting enough appropriate fats. Fats can also help you feel satiated longer after a meal and keep you from consuming more junk an hour after you finish eating.

Many of my clients are very excited to learn that foods, like butter, whole eggs or heavy cream, can actually be beneficial to their health and aid in weight loss. When it comes to fats, depending on your body chemistry at the cellular level, certain fats will help you as much as any supplement could, while other specific fats could push you in the wrong direction. In chapter seven I teach how to look at a few simple measurements to figure out if you have any imbalances that could benefit from consuming specific fats. If you're balanced, most healthy fats can benefit you greatly.

The important factor that confuses the issue is that digestion needs to be working correctly for your body to be able to process fats correctly. Without proper bile flow, you can't emulsify those fats so that the body can use them. The Beet Flow supplement I talked about before will help improve that. This is why a diet that is higher in fats doesn't work for everyone. If you don't have the bile flow to process fats correctly, increasing your fat intake could lead to gaining weight. But if you do have good bile flow, increasing your appropriate fats can speed up weight loss greatly; and avoiding fats can restrict weight loss altogether for some of you.

Here is the shortlist of fats that many people avoid but can actually aid in weight loss if used with the correct body chemistry:

Egg yolks
Butter
Coconut oil
Heavy cream
Olive oil
Animal fats
Avocado
Nuts

Many dieters also eliminate good fats and replace them with products that boast to be healthier options, even though the replacement products create more fat storage than the version of that food that they are trying to replace. Things like:

Vegetable oils
Butter-replacement spreads
Fat-free dairy products
Fat-free baked goods

When manufactures reduce fats in these products, they add chemicals and artificial sweeteners in order to keep flavor. These chemicals are the things your body doesn't recognize as food; therefore the chemicals will often get stored in fat cells. Oops.

Mineral Levels And Cravings

Remember, this is the formula:
If minerals are too low, raising sugars can help.
If sugars are too low, raising minerals can help.

Since raising sugars will also raise insulin levels and cause weight gain, the trick is to look at your physiology to see if you are a person who needs to raise your minerals or not. If you have high blood pressure, this is an indication that your body is not correctly handling the minerals you currently have. So, raising mineral levels is not a good option for you and, in some cases, could be dangerous. However, if your blood pressure is low, raising your mineral levels could give you a new lease on life, health, and especially weight loss.

In chapter seven you'll learn how to test your blood pressure to get a sense of your mineral levels, whether high or low. If your mineral levels are high and you want to improve cravings, you'll likely want to focus more on digestion and including more good fats. But if your blood pressure is low, you'll likely want to put a lot of attention into what I'm going to explain here.

If digestion has been poor for years, the body could be very depleted when it comes to mineral reserves. Increasing the minerals available to the body can make a huge difference in how every part of that body operates. It can also reduce how often your body screams at you for some Nutter Butters.

If you're using supplements to improve digestion, more minerals will be brought in from the food you're eating. On that same front, increasing use of unrefined salt (like sea salt) can be a life-changing step for someone with low blood pressure. Chapter eight outlines all the numbers to look for while determining if your blood pressure is high or low. If your blood pressure is low, don't be afraid of sea salt. We're taught to avoid salt because many years ago the doctor told our Uncle Phil it's going to kill him. Yes, if you have high blood pressure, you certainly may want to correct it before you start to add salt. But as a society, we have taken advice directed at those with high blood pressure and applied that advice to everyone. Even to those who REALLY need that salt. You'll read more about salt in chapter twelve. Just know that I've seen more clients reduce their cravings and improve a variety of health issues from simply adding sea salt than any other suggestion I offer.

Blackstrap molasses is another excellent source of minerals (the higher the potassium per tablespoon, the better). Molasses has some sugar content as well, so you want to be mindful of that. Yet using a half teaspoon in a protein shake, cup of hot tea, or even cooked into a stir fry, can be an excellent way to boost your mineral intake each day.

In chapter sixteen I talk more about supplements that can help lift minerals as well, but unrefined salt and blackstrap molasses are the best places to start if you have low blood pressure.

Note: If you are on blood pressure medication, that drug will artificially keep your blood pressure low. So, don't look at that low blood pressure reading and think you need more mineral. If you're on blood pressure medication and now have a blood pressure reading that could be considered too low, you might want to talk to your doctor about lowering the dosage of your medication. Keep in mind that I'm not telling you to lower your medication. You need to consult your doctor to make a move like that.

Soil And Minerals

It is believed that, as humans, we are hardwired for foods that are sweet. You see, when food is the way it's supposed to be, where we find sweet is also where we used to find a lot of minerals—like in fruit, for example. These minerals are what help us process the sugars in these sweet foods. The majority of fruit grown today is lacking the mineral needed to handle the sugars contained in that fruit. That is why fruit is often not the healthy choice that it once was. The result can be people thinking that they're making a healthy selection when they're really just eating a candy bar that grew on a tree.

To make matters worse, the manufacturing industry takes a food like corn and processes the minerals out of it while producing some type of corn flake or snack foods. First, they take out the germ. Next, they coat the remaining complex carbs with sugar to make it delicious and appealing to our senses. The brain sees this sweet product as having an abundance of mineral. This triggers the brain's happy receptors letting the body know that nutrients are on the way. The brain says, "You need mineral badly; now eat a bucket of this stuff." An hour and a half after eating an entire bucket of sweet, nutritionally void "non-food," the person is looking for something else to eat. The body got ripped off and didn't receive what it thought it was getting, so it starts to look for something sweet that can bring in the mineral that it needs.

Beyond the processing of food, the real trouble with today's food source shows up when processing begins with the soil. People talk a lot about how the real problem is the American soil and how it has no mineral left in it. The Italians have been growing tomatoes for over 5,000 years, yet they still grow a good tomato. America has been farming for what, three hundred years? And we can't grow a tomato that tastes like anything anymore. You can see that it's red, but if you've ever talked to anyone who has eaten produce in other countries, they will tell you, "Over there, it actually has flavor in it."

The American soil is not the problem, it is the American farming methods. Minerals need to be in the soil in order for minerals to be able to make it into the plant. However, it's the bacteria in the soil that allows the mineral to make that jump from the dirt to the plant, and then into the fruit of that plant. The bacteria is the life of that soil. When you fertilize with chemical and high phosphate fertilizers, you kill the bacteria and the mineral can't make the jump into the plant.

The problem is this: We now have brilliant scientists who have figured out how to engineer the seed so that it no longer requires minerals to produce an apparent crop. Why do I say 'apparent' crop? Because that's what the crops are: Produce that appears before you, even though it is void of mineral. Crops aren't even weighed anymore; they are sold by the bushel, which means they are sold by the size and not the weight. Mineral is what makes a crop weigh more, so there is no financial punishment for a farmer who sells a crop void of significant nutritional value. Are you following the path our food takes? We have the farmer "processing" the very soil and seed that our food comes from, then the product manufacturers "process" that produce into something that doesn't resemble food at all, and then we pray over it like the miracle of nature had anything to do with making it? Oops. That's why it's becoming so important to use good supplements that are appropriate for your body. This is becoming the only way to ensure that you're getting the nutrients you really need since our food supply is slowly turning into nothing more than something to chew on.

Is There Crack In These Snack Cakes?

Are you starting to understand why these processed junk foods can be so addicting? Food mad scientists have figured out how to make processed foods taste like there is nutrition inside. If your body is depleted of needed minerals and other nutrients, and you eat foods that send the brain a signal that states, "Here comes the nutrition you've been missing," of course the body will be tricked into wanting more. When artificial sweeteners are even sweeter than foods found in nature, consuming these sweet tastes can jack up your cravings even more.

These chemical sweeteners should be avoided even more than sugar when trying to kill cravings.

We are also drawn to salty and fatty flavors because in nature, these flavors are attached to the nutrients we need the most. In nature, sweet, salty and fatty foods are filled with minerals, vitamins, proteins and fats that our bodies need to function. The obesity problem in this country is not an issue of slackers who have no self control at the dinner table. These are just people who are having their innate, hard-wired system used against them by the food manufacturers. Some of these food manufacturers make the people who make cigarettes look like upstanding citizens. At least the cigarette folks tell you right on the package that their product is not good for you. There are other factors often involved in cravings and obesity, but helping people realize that the food they are eating is really more of a "non-food" and doesn't count as nutrition can be a big step in the right direction.

When the nutrients never show up, the body isn't going to change the innate functionality it has been operating on for eons. The body is not going to say, "I guess sweet taste no longer equates to a good source of minerals." Our bodies have been operating this way for thousands of years. We've only been bastardizing our food supply for a few decades. This means you should not count on evolution to correct your cravings.

You do have one option, however. You can stop eating the junk. Just because some evil genius has discovered how to make his snack cakes more addictive than crack doesn't mean that you are required to continue supporting his new speed boat. His desire to be rich does not need to win out over your desire to be healthy.

The difficulty of eliminating these foods will come down to your mineral content. If you can give your body what it really needs, your body will stop screaming for this junk that mimics the nutrients your body is searching for. This can give you the edge over food that may have kept you captive in the past. With your knowledge of why you crave these foods and what you can do to reduce those cravings, it can be your turn to win. I wonder if you'll get a speed boat too.

Low & Medium-Carb Foods

When it comes to weight loss, an important goal should be to eliminate cravings and bingeing. Once you take care of those two issues, the rest is pretty easy. You already learned that correcting digestion in order to get more mineral into the system can reduce cravings and the need to binge.

But sometimes more mineral isn't enough. With some people who have low blood pressure, you can add a lot more mineral and they will still have low resources because they have been depleting the body's reserves for so long. In some cases, these people seem to have a malfunction that causes them to pee out their minerals as fast as they are ingested. These individuals will often benefit from consuming more carbs, at least in the beginning, while these folks do the work to bring mineral levels up naturally.

At the same time, we know that increasing carbs is going to reduce the speed at which you lose weight. Yes, you can lose weight much faster by consuming fewer carbs. However, if you don't have many mineral reserves, I would prefer to see you achieve a slow, gradual weight loss. If you try to lose six pounds in a week by eating very few carbs, you may end up snapping and bingeing on a box of doughnuts that makes you gain seven pounds.

This is where medium-carb foods come in. By selecting foods that can provide more carbs, without spiking insulin levels as much as high-carb choices might, you can keep your cravings down and your sanity up, and still lose weight.

The type of carbs will be important. You still need to avoid all sugar and starchy carbs that will spike insulin levels too high. That means avoiding bread, rice, pasta, potatoes, etc. If you consume fruit, try to stick to lower glycemic fruits like berries or maybe half an apple.

Low-Carb Examples

A low-carb meal would contain between 0 and 15 active carbs.
- Spinach omelet using three whole eggs, with real butter and two turkey sausage links.
- Grilled chicken caesar salad without croutons.

- Two baked chicken legs with a side of broccoli.

Medium-Carb Examples

A medium-carb meal would contain between 16 and 25 active carbs.
- Lettuce wrap with grilled chicken, snap peas, hummus, and butternut squash.
- Greek yogurt with berries.
- Protein shake with a teaspoon of blackstrap molasses.
- Grilled Salmon with lentils and broccoli.
- A small apple with almond butter.

If you're already improving digestion and adding unrefined salt or other mineral sources and cravings are still strong, the goal could be to have 16-25 active carbs per meal for three meals of the day. Going higher than 25 active carbs could cause your insulin to spike too high and then your blood sugar will drop too low and you will crave sugar or carbs big time. So, the trick is to get in more carbs without spiking insulin levels too high.

Once you do add a few carbs and can stop the cravings and bingeing, you can begin trying to remove most of your carbs from dinner. Stopping carbs after 3:00 PM will allow you to start dropping weight.

If removing most carbs from dinner becomes easy, you can do this every day. You might want to try removing carbs from dinner for just one or two days in a row and then having some medium-carbs for dinner again on the third day. If that goes well, try to go for more days in a row.

Once low-carb dinners are easy, try removing carbs from lunch as well in the same manner. Maybe you try that for only a day or so at a time at first to make sure cravings don't come back.

Keep reducing medium-carb meals until you can do a whole day with no medium-carb meals. Just don't try to do this every day because you don't need to lose weight that quickly. But if you can drop the carbs on every meal other than breakfast for 3-5 days of the week, you will likely begin to lose weight.

When you want to be aggressive and lose weight faster, try reducing more carbs. If any cravings come on again or any thoughts of binges, eat a medium-carb food as quickly as possible and go back to more carbs in the day. (Keep in mind that you should still be doing the work to raise mineral levels as you learn to reduce carbs.)

You'll need to look at labels and watch the active carb content of what you're eating. Try to find foods with carbs that fit the numbers you're looking for.

Don't worry about a daily limit on carbs. This method can be too restrictive. Just try to give yourself long periods of the day where you have no insulin spikes. Keeping insulin down is where your weight loss will come from. That's why no insulin spikes after 3:00 PM is so effective. It gives you the rest of the afternoon and the whole night to burn fat.

To find lists of low-carb and medium-carb foods, go to www.DoneWithThatBooks.com and click on BOOK TOOLS > LOW-CARB CHARTS or MEDIUM-CARB CHARTS.

Wha'd He Say?

In this chapter, you learned:

- Cravings can be reduced or eliminated by improving digestion and finding other ways to give your body what it really needs.
- If blood pressure is low, finding ways to bring up the mineral content in the system can reduce cravings. Unrefined salt and blackstrap molasses can be great places to start.
- Consuming appropriate fats can reduce cravings.
- Most processed foods are scientifically designed to make you feel better by telling your body that nutrition is on the way—even though it's not. It will, however, trigger the happy receptors in your brain, making you want to eat more of this junk. Because of this, the goal should be to bring in more of the minerals and nutrients your body truly needs so you can feel better without the junk.
- Using medium-carb foods strategically can help reduce cravings for those who have a low mineral content.

CHAPTER SEVEN

Simple Self-Testing

You're about to learn how to run very simple physiological tests on your body. The information you gain from these tests will direct you to nutritional choices and lifestyle changes that could help you reach your goals the easiest. However, I'm going to share only the simple tests here. If you find that you would like to run additional tests and gain even more information, you can follow the intermediate self-testing instructions in Appendix B.

You have an opportunity here to begin understanding how your specific body is operating. You may be able to recognize imbalances that you are experiencing and you may even find food, nutrition or lifestyle changes that could help improve those imbalances. Just be sure to understand that the body is very complicated. In most cases, if a person is serious about improving a severe symptom, condition, or something even more serious, that individual is going to need help from a professional who has a firm grasp on these foundational principles. So, don't try to be a hero and figure it all out yourself. There really is no reason to show off in that way, and you will much more likely create added frustration for yourself. I'm going to teach you what to look at and where you can find tools to chart your progress and monitor your changes on your own. I'm also going to show you where you can find help when you need it. Be sure you understand how much time and effort you will save by finding a professional to help you along.

It's important to understand that people need to take responsibility for their own health. Most people will not be able to simply take a few supplements, or remove a few foods from their diet, and correct every issue that may have been developing for the last two or three decades.

You will, however, be able to watch your chemistry and see if you are moving in the right direction, even before you might notice any changes in how you feel. For many, improved chemistry is often enough to keep them on track long enough to reap the rewards.

This approach is much different from only treating a symptom. The medical world is not the only place where practitioners treat off of symptom. Most natural practitioners work off of symptoms as well. They just use natural substances to improve those symptoms instead of drugs, but they are still pigeonholing a client into a "diagnosis" based on the symptoms. When working in this manner, a practitioner might as well be asking the clients to throw darts at a "diagnosis dart board." At least with this option, clients might leave the doctor's office with a stuffed animal.

However, when natural practitioners do guess correctly, a natural approach often doesn't bring about an immediate "drug-like" response. Therefore, the client stops or moves on to the next big thing.

When looking to help your body correct its own issues, keep in mind that this process will take much longer than the 4-6 hours it often takes for a drug to kick in. In nature, things that happen fast are often bad things. The best things happen slowly. A flower doesn't wake up and go, "BAM!!!" open. The flower opens very slowly and gradually. The sun doesn't just appear out of nowhere in full force. That would freak us out every single time. The sun rises gradually, just as it sets, just as the grass grows and the seasons change. Let your body do the same. If you're looking to "fix" a problem by Friday because you don't want it to interfere with the big square dance you hope to attend, you're going to find yourself very frustrated—not only because you really need a better social life if a square dance is your big event, but also because you're setting yourself up for failure if you believe you can change the agriculture of your body in a few days. You can't.

Data Tracking Sheet

In this section you will find a *Data Tracking Sheet*. You can also go to the site, www.DoneWithThatBooks.com and download a free PDF to print so you won't have to mark up your pretty book. This will allow you to keep a binder of your progress so you can track your results and see patterns. You will also have that information available in case you decide to seek help from a professional. Click on the link BOOK TOOLS to download the *Data Tracking Sheet*. While you're at it, you can also download the *Basic Imbalance Guide*, as I cover that form in chapter eight.

On the top right corner of the *Data Tracking Sheet*, you will see colored boxes that are used when testing your urine with an 11-parameter strip. These strips are used as part of the intermediate testing procedures outlined in Appendix B. You won't need to use those colored boxes unless you decide you want to collect more information about your chemistry.

URINE TEST STRIP

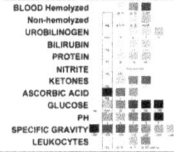

BLOOD Hemolyzed
Non-hemolyzed
UROBILINOGEN
BILIRUBIN
PROTEIN
NITRITE
KETONES
ASCORBIC ACID
GLUCOSE
PH
SPECIFIC GRAVITY
LEUKOCYTES

Date_____ Time_____	Date_____ Time_____	Date_____ Time_____	Date_____ Time_____
Well-Being_____	Well-Being_____	Well-Being_____	Well-Being_____
Urine pH _____	Urine pH _____	Urine pH _____	Urine pH _____
Saliva pH _____	Saliva pH _____	Saliva pH _____	Saliva pH _____
Breath Rate _____	Breath Rate _____	Breath Rate _____	Breath Rate _____
Breat Hold _____	Breat Hold _____	Breat Hold _____	Breat Hold _____
Resting Standing	**Resting Standing**	**Resting Standing**	**Resting Standing**
Blood Pressure (Systolic) _____ _____	Blood Pressure (Systolic) _____ _____	Blood Pressure (Systolic) _____ _____	Blood Pressure (Systolic) _____ _____
Blood Pressure (Diastolic) _____ _____	Blood Pressure (Diastolic) _____ _____	Blood Pressure (Diastolic) _____ _____	Blood Pressure (Diastolic) _____ _____
Pulse _____ _____	Pulse _____ _____	Pulse _____ _____	Pulse _____ _____

Date_____ Time_____	Date_____ Time_____	Date_____ Time_____	Date_____ Time_____
Well-Being_____	Well-Being_____	Well-Being_____	Well-Being_____
Urine pH _____	Urine pH _____	Urine pH _____	Urine pH _____
Saliva pH _____	Saliva pH _____	Saliva pH _____	Saliva pH _____
Breath Rate _____	Breath Rate _____	Breath Rate _____	Breath Rate _____
Breat Hold _____	Breat Hold _____	Breat Hold _____	Breat Hold _____
Resting Standing	**Resting Standing**	**Resting Standing**	**Resting Standing**
Blood Pressure (Systolic) _____ _____	Blood Pressure (Systolic) _____ _____	Blood Pressure (Systolic) _____ _____	Blood Pressure (Systolic) _____ _____
Blood Pressure (Diastolic) _____ _____	Blood Pressure (Diastolic) _____ _____	Blood Pressure (Diastolic) _____ _____	Blood Pressure (Diastolic) _____ _____
Pulse _____ _____	Pulse _____ _____	Pulse _____ _____	Pulse _____ _____

Date_____ Time_____	Date_____ Time_____	Date_____ Time_____	Date_____ Time_____
Well-Being_____	Well-Being_____	Well-Being_____	Well-Being_____
Urine pH _____	Urine pH _____	Urine pH _____	Urine pH _____
Saliva pH _____	Saliva pH _____	Saliva pH _____	Saliva pH _____
Breath Rate _____	Breath Rate _____	Breath Rate _____	Breath Rate _____
Breat Hold _____	Breat Hold _____	Breat Hold _____	Breat Hold _____
Resting Standing	**Resting Standing**	**Resting Standing**	**Resting Standing**
Blood Pressure (Systolic) _____ _____	Blood Pressure (Systolic) _____ _____	Blood Pressure (Systolic) _____ _____	Blood Pressure (Systolic) _____ _____
Blood Pressure (Diastolic) _____ _____	Blood Pressure (Diastolic) _____ _____	Blood Pressure (Diastolic) _____ _____	Blood Pressure (Diastolic) _____ _____
Pulse _____ _____	Pulse _____ _____	Pulse _____ _____	Pulse _____ _____

The Coalition

There is an international association called *The Coalition for Health Education*. This private, nonprofit association spans the planet and consists of doctors, health coaches, nutritionists, a wide variety of other types of natural health professionals and members of the general public who want to learn more about natural health and how the body really works. When readers come to www.DoneWithThatBooks.com looking for a health coach who can help them better understand the ideas that are taught in this book, we send them to *The Coalition* to find a professional in their area.

We have also made arrangements with this private association to allow our readers to become members without sponsorship from a professional health coach. *The Coalition* has an advanced website that was put in place to help health coaches educate their clients and monitor the progress of their client's chemistry. As those clients input the numbers from their self-tests into the website, the health coach can help them make nutritional adjustments according to their chemistry. However, even if you are not working with a health coach, as one of my readers, you can register as a member of the site, which will grant you access to all of your own advanced monitoring and tracking tools. I helped them put together many of the systems they use today so they have given my readers the hook-up. As you input the results of your self-tests into the system, you can watch the changes over time in the site's dynamic graphing systems. You can even keep a food journal to which your self-test results will transfer automatically so you can see how different foods affect your chemistry and how you feel. You will also find charts that can show you where your chemistry is now, and what foods can help push you in the right direction if you are imbalanced.

It is an amazing tool. The best part is that $20 per year will cover your membership dues and there is no extra charge to use the tools on the website. As an added benefit, if you decide that you need the help of a professional in your area, *The Coalition* can attach your account to a local health coach who can then see how your chemistry has been moving while you were working on your own.

The downloadable *Data Tracking Sheet* found at www.DoneWithThatBooks.com is an adequate way to keep tabs on your chemistry; but if you really want to see the whole picture by using the graphs and other tools, *The Coalition* is the way to go. If you have an Internet connection and can afford $20 for the year, you'll want to take advantage of this arrangement. It has been a very helpful tool for *Done With That* readers. For the remainder of this book, it may sound like I'm assuming you are using the tools on *The Coalition* website because I feel like they can really help you see into your numbers and better understand your chemistry. I assume that you are using them because they are helpful tools that will make this process much easier. You can call me lazy if you like, but I tend to move toward methods that make my life easier. Monitoring measurements can validate you are going in the right direction. This gives you the discernment to stay on course. It's easier to keep doing the right thing when your own measurements make the process become more objective instead of subjective.

Investing in your own health is as important as taking the time to read about it. Though improving the actual cause of a problem can take work and sometimes money, I always tell my clients that sooner or later you're going to pay for your health. You can pay now and the money you spend will go toward preventative measures and long-term improvement, or you can pay later and those funds will go toward holding you together or trying to repair something that has gone horribly wrong. We all pay, the option of *when* is up to us.

"If you ignore your health long enough it WILL go away."
- My Pen Pal

You can go directly to www.OurCoalition.org and click on Self-Monitoring Registration to take the tour of all the site has to offer.

Let's Get To Testing...

If you haven't acquired the necessary testing materials that I talked about at the end of chapter one, are you procrastinating, or are you just a really fast reader? Now is the time to have those tools so you can see where your chemistry is before I talk more about each imbalance. It's easy to listen to symptoms that go along with each imbalance and say, "Oh yeah, that's totally me, I must have that imbalance." But that's the wrong way to look at your individuality.

Let's say that you desperately need to go to Hallmark to pick up a card from their "I accidentally called my mother-in-law fat" section. When you get to the mall, the first thing you look for is the directory. Once you find Hallmark on the directory, what do you do next? That's right, you look for the "You Are Here" red dot. If you don't know where you are, how are you going to find where you need to go? Testing yourself is finding the red dot.

Some of you may not need to run all of these tests. Many of you will be able to run just a few procedures and the results will be so clear, it will give you an obvious path to follow on your weight loss journey. Others will need to use more tests, and some readers will need to seek the help of a professional who can look at other parameters of their chemistry. Many of these professionals have special equipment or software that can supply information about your chemistry beyond the methods I can provide in this book.

Simple Testing Procedures

It can be helpful to perform the simple self-tests on a regular basis, at least in the beginning. They are very simple and can easily fit into your current daily activities once you make them a habit. I like to see people run most of these tests at least twice a week for the first few weeks so you can get an idea of where your chemistry truly is. This becomes the "You Are Here" dot on the mall directory. However, because I am teaching you how to look at only a few parameters, it is a good idea to run these simple tests four or five times in the first week. This gives you more of a video image of how your body is operating instead of a snapshot.

Simply perform these tests and mark the results on your *Data Tracking Sheet* or input them into the Progress Charts on *The Coalition*. On the tracking sheet, there are data boxes for twelve different testings. Each time you test yourself, just add the date and time to the top of one of the boxes and input your numbers. You see spaces for water intake, urine pH, saliva pH, breath rate and breath hold. We left a blank space below breath hold for those who may need to check their fasting glucose daily.

Below breath hold you can input your blood pressure reading, which will include your systolic blood pressure (the top number), diastolic blood pressure (the number below the systolic), and your pulse (the bottom number on most automatic blood pressure cuffs).

The water intake space on the *Data Tracking Sheet* should be filled in according to how much water you have had up to the point of testing for that day. This information can be useful in helping you understand why your numbers are where they are. If your blood pressure is much lower than normal (optimal reading being 120/80), you may be able to see that you have consumed more water than normal on that day, which has washed away too many minerals and brought down your blood pressure. In any case, viewing your numbers in relation to your water intake can be helpful.

Depending on the issues you are trying to improve, you might check only your blood pressure, breath rate, or pHs on some days. That is acceptable and any information is helpful in my book. (Wait a minute; this is my book, so I guess that goes without saying.) Always put the date and time at the top of each box and fill in test results from that time only. It's okay to leave blanks when you don't run all of the tests. When you use the tracking tools on *The Coalition*, you will also have the option to input only a pH or blood pressure reading if that is all you test that day.

pH of Urine and Saliva

It is best if you don't test your urine pH right when you wake up. The first morning urine test, while being a valid test, takes greater discretion to sort out the results because you are unloading the previous day's "metabolic debt," those acids you accumulated through the previous day. Understanding the results of that first morning test is quite complicated and I don't cover that in this book. Testing your urine and saliva pH either just before lunch or just before dinner (ideally at least two hours since you have eaten any food) will be an easier test to discern what the numbers are showing.

Urine pH

Hold the test strip in your urine stream for a second and read the result against the color chart found on the packaging. If the chart reads in half-point increments, and your reading is between two colors, make an estimate for your reading. For example, if the color on your pH strip falls between 6 and 6.5, make a guess and say 6.3 or wherever you think it lands. Just pick a number and don't say "really green" or "very yellow," because that is too subjective. Pick a number; you are simply looking for a range. If the actual reading is off by a little bit, that's okay. You won't be using NASA equipment here and you're not going to get an exact reading. You just want to be able to see, "Is it high or is it low? How high or low is it?" So, don't drive yourself nuts and think that you have to pull out the magnifying glass and read the strip under indoor lighting that mimics the sun at high noon. Just look at the pee on the strip and mark it down.

Saliva pH

Try not to drink or have anything in your mouth for 20 minutes before testing, and ideally you want to wait approximately two hours after eating. Testing your saliva at the same time as your urine will keep everything simple. Don't use the same strip for both—it makes me sad that I feel like I need to explain that (however I do know one person who takes a pair of scissors and splits the strip long ways to get twice as many measurements out of a pack). Bring up a little saliva between your lips and run the test strip across your lips and through the saliva. Read against the chart right away. Timing is important. The CO_2 in your saliva will out-gas into the atmosphere. The reading will often rise the longer you wait to read it. Because of this, it is best to read the saliva as soon as you moisten the strip or you will have a less accurate reading. With urine, it is not as important to read against the chart right away.

Blood Pressure

To test your resting blood pressure, lie down and relax for two minutes or so. Perform the test on your left arm according to the directions for your blood pressure cuff. If you are using an automatic cuff, it will likely display three numbers, usually in this configuration: The top number is the systolic pressure (measure of blood pressure while the heart is beating). The middle number is the diastolic pressure (measure of blood pressure while the heart is relaxed). The bottom number is your pulse. If it is difficult for you to lie down for the reading, you can take this test in a seated, resting position.

On the Data Tracking Sheet you will see spaces for both resting and standing blood pressures. You will only use the standing blood pressure slots if you move up to the intermediate self-tests found in Appendix B.

Breath Rate

This can be difficult to test on yourself. When you're conscious of what you're doing, you might adjust your breathing, even subconsciously. Anytime you can, get someone else to count this for you so you can let your mind wander to other things and just breathe normally. Doing so will likely provide a more accurate reading. If you don't have that option, just try to count your breaths while breathing as normally as possible. Lie down and relax. Try to think of other things so that you breathe normally. Start your timer and count the number of times you inhale in 30 seconds. Double that number for the number of breaths per minute. Just be sure you don't count an inhale as one and an exhale as two. Count only the inhales. I like to continue for the entire minute to see if I get the same number the last 30 seconds as I did the first. If not, I may average the two. My preference is to use an egg timer, so you can set it for one minute and the timer will count down to zero, allowing you to count your inhales without having to worry about the timer since it will beep when the minute is up. This can be the easiest way to perform this test if you don't have someone to help you.

Breath Hold Time

Sit comfortably. Take three full, deep breaths in and out. Near the end of the fourth inhale, start your stopwatch or timer and hold your breath as long as you can. Don't pass out or turn blue or turn this into a contest you have to win. Guys will typically try to hold their breath longer, as if this is some type of macho sign. Not once have I noticed a girl across a room, walked up to her and said, "Hey, watch how long I can hold my breath." So guys, just know that this is not as cool as you may think it to be. That being said, do hold your breath as long as you comfortably can. It's best not to look at the stopwatch while you're holding your breath. If you do, you may be inclined to turn it into a competition and hold your breath longer than you normally would.

Bonus Test - Blood Glucose

If you have a lot of weight to lose, it's very important to know where your blood sugar levels are. Even if you are not extremely overweight, you could still be diabetic or moving in that direction and have no idea. If you can test your fasting blood glucose at least once, you can rule out high blood sugar from the picture. If your blood sugar is high and you don't know it, you will have a very hard time seeing any major weight loss results.

To get your fasting glucose, test before breakfast, before you drink anything other than water, and, if possible, before you brush your teeth. When you want to check your fasting glucose, it's best to leave the glucometer out where you will see it first thing in the morning so you won't forget.

If your results fall into the normal range of 70 - 90, you probably won't need to perform this test very often. If your results are over 100, you're going to want to monitor this regularly until the reading comes into range.

It is important that you wash your hands prior to testing so residues from lotions, etc. don't affect the test results. Most glucometers will come with a lancing device and a few disposable lancets. This lancing device is used to poke the skin of your finger, allowing a small amount of blood to emerge. Insert a new disposable lancet into your lancing device. (Never re-use lancets. You may also be using an all-in-one disposable lancet where you just remove the plastic safety cover from the needle, cock the lancet and push a button to set it off while holding the tip to your finger.) Prick your finger and allow the blood to make a small bubble. (It's best not to squeeze your finger, if you can avoid doing so, since that may give you a lower blood sugar reading.) Depending on your glucometer, either drip the blood on top of the test strip or place the test strip up against the drop of blood and it will sip the blood up into the strip like a straw. The glucometer will normally calculate the measurement for a few moments before it displays your blood glucose number.

Easy Peasy

That's it. Your testing is done. In chapter eight I teach you what these simple test results can indicate in regard to your body and your physiology. You're about to know a whole bunch of stuff. And when you talk about it, you'll be able to use words that are fancier than "stuff."

Wha'd He Say?

In this chapter, you learned:

- If your chemistry or health situation is complicated, get help from a professional who understands this work. You will still be a participant in your own health.
- Correcting the actual underlying cause of a problem will take longer than the four hours it takes for a drug to kick in. Be patient.
- Go to www.OurCoalition.org to register as a member and gain access to tracking tools that will help you reach your goals.
- Try to take any tests at least two hours after a meal.
- Testing yourself is the key to understanding your next move. How do you know what to do next if you don't know where you are now?

CHAPTER EIGHT

Understanding Your Biological Individuality

Intro To Imbalances

This will be the most sciency chapter. You can tell how complicated it will be by my use of such a technical word as "sciency." Don't let the technical aspects scare you away. I promise to talk in stories and analogies as often as possible. It's true that many readers have learned enough to lose an incredible amount of weight by the time they reach this chapter. Many of you could have easily stopped reading after chapter three and still had the ability to see results if you followed the guidelines on correcting digestion. However, if you've ever had a diet not work for you, you're about to understand why. Learning how to look at your own biological individuality can uncover which foods are best for you... not your neighbor or your brother or even that dreamy kid in all the vampire movies... You.

Beyond digestive issues that may need attention, there are ten main imbalances that can occur in the body. To simplify this book, I cover only six of these imbalances because they are the ones that most commonly contribute to weight gain. Understanding your optimal food choices is valuable enough to wade through some science. With that in mind, push through anything that is a little complicated and I promise I'll get back to the simple stuff in chapter ten. This is my favorite part but I tried my best not to blab on for hours. For those who want to dig in deeper, you can read Appendix C where I cover all ten imbalances. To learn about the pioneers who created the work that makes up the bulk of what I cover in this series, read *Those Who Paved the Way* in Appendix D.

I first want to teach you how to look at your self-test numbers that you learned how to find in chapter seven. In that way, you'll know which imbalances you need to pay close attention to when I explain how each imbalance can contribute to weight gain in its own way. For now, I'll give you a very brief introduction to each imbalance. Each imbalance has a polar opposite so I go over them in pairs.

Electrolyte Excess and Electrolyte Deficiency Imbalances

These imbalances can indicate the level of electrolytes in the system. An Electrolyte Excess Imbalance would show that there are too many minerals in the system and a possible inability for the body to remove junk, often resulting in high blood pressure. Almost 50% of Americans fall into this category. Those dealing with hypertension and cardiovascular disease are often experiencing an Electrolyte Excess Imbalance.

An Electrolyte Deficiency Imbalance would show a lack of mineral in the system, leaving the body without enough resources to function properly. This is a common imbalance for those with uncontrollable cravings. Depression, vertigo, menstrual or muscle cramps, or insomnia are often seen with an Electrolyte Deficiency Imbalance. PLEASE remember that these symptoms can also be caused by other imbalances for completely different reasons. Don't assume you have an imbalance because you have a symptom that often shows up with that imbalance (I will say this at least nine more times).

Anabolic and Catabolic Imbalances

These imbalances describe cellular permeability. Whether or not the body is in the breaking down (catabolic) or building up (anabolic) phase is a major focus when it comes to these two imbalances. Knowing cellular permeability can give you system-wide information instead of the tunnel vision that symptoms normally provide

Fat Burner and Carb Burner Imbalances

The body is designed to burn both fats and glucose, generally speaking. Some individuals get stuck burning more fats than glucose, or vice versa. If one of these imbalances shows as a result of your self-tests, you would likely be burning predominantly fat or glucose. This is key information for those who wish to increase their energy or lose weight.

The point I drive home throughout this book is this: With just about any symptom (like excess body fat), there can be multiple causes. Some symptoms can be more serious than others. Some may be easier to improve. Some may not apply to you at all. It's likely that I cover topics that will have you thinking, "What the heck does this have to do with my fat butt? Why can't this idiot just get to the point?" Remember that this book is about improving health and not about fighting or beating one problem. The body is a complex machine, even more complex than an Etch-a-Sketch. (I'm really good at making the stairs.) Many issues and imbalances can have layers of causes that all need to be addressed. In that same manner, one little imbalance can throw five or six systems out of whack; and, if you can improve that one imbalance, all kinds of craziness can go back to normal and excess fat can melt away.

I am about to cover how symptoms can be used as a piece of data, but that DOES NOT mean that the symptoms are the data. If you and I were standing in my kitchen talking about this right now, I would shake you just to make sure you were listening to me. I also really like to shake people while I try to make a funny point just to see if I can get away with it. I have a very limited number of people punch me in the neck when I do that, so it's always fun to see what I can get away with. In any case, pretend I just shook you so that the point about symptoms and jumping to conclusions sinks in.

With chapter seven teaching you how to run simple tests, the next step is for me to help you understand how these numbers can be translated into imbalances. In other words, now we can look at how whacked you really are and why your fat won't just leave you alone and go away. Even though one of the goals of this book is to sway you from living your life through symptoms, you can still use symptoms to further understand where your body chemistry may be going awry. Symptoms become more meaningful when they are seen in a context of biological measurement. With that in mind, be certain you don't look at a symptom that is sometimes associated with an imbalance and assume you must have that imbalance. Use the numbers as your main reference point.

Imbalance Guide

On the next page, you see a copy of the *Basic Imbalance Guide* (referred to as *Imbalance Guide* for the rest of the book). If you didn't download a copy when you printed off your *Data Tracking Sheet*, you can do that now. Go to our website, www.DoneWithThatBooks.com. Just click on BOOK TOOLS and BASIC IMBALANCE GUIDE. I also include here a sample *Imbalance Guide* that has been filled out. This will give you a visual of how specific results can help to determine whether or not you should circle an imbalance that needs correction or underline an imbalance that may need a little boost in the right direction.

IMBALANCE GUIDE

Name: _____   Date: _____ Time: _____

Electrolyte Status

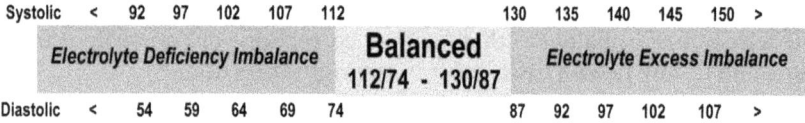

Systolic	<	92	97	102	107	112		130	135	140	145	150	>

Electrolyte Deficiency Imbalance | **Balanced** 112/74 - 130/87 | *Electrolyte Excess Imbalance*

Diastolic	<	54	59	64	69	74		87	92	97	102	107	>

Circle Your Breath Rate

Less Than 10 See Appendix C	10 11 12 13 14 15 16 17 18 19 20	More Than 20 See Appendix C

Breath Hold Time = _____ Seconds

Catabolic/Anabolic Validators

Catabolic	Anabolic
__ Urine pH < 6.1	Urine pH > 6.3 __
__ Saliva pH > 6.9	Saliva pH < 6.6 __
__ Oliguria	Polyuria __
__ Soft/Loose Stool	Hard Stool / Constipation __
__ Wake Easily	Difficult to Rise __
__ High Debris in Urine	Low Debris in Urine __
__ Migraines	Anxiety __

pH Chart

Urine

8.0
May Push urine pH down
Monitor to Validate

Organ Meats
Vitamin C as ascorbic acid

7.5

7.0

6.5

5.8 ~ 6.3
Optimal Zone When
Breath Rate is 16~20

6.0

5.5
Butter
Coconut Oil

May Push urine pH up
Monitor to Validate
5.0

= My Optimal Zones

Saliva

May Push Saliva pH down
Monitor to Validate

Sauerkraut
Yogurt
Betaine HCL
Cayenne Pepper Capsules
Lemon in Water

5.5 - 6.0
Optimal Zone When
Breath Rate is 10~15

Vitamin B12
Digestive Enzymes
CoQ10

Cottage Cheese
Corn Meal
Lima Beans
Buckwheat
Squash

May Push Saliva pH up
Monitor to Validate

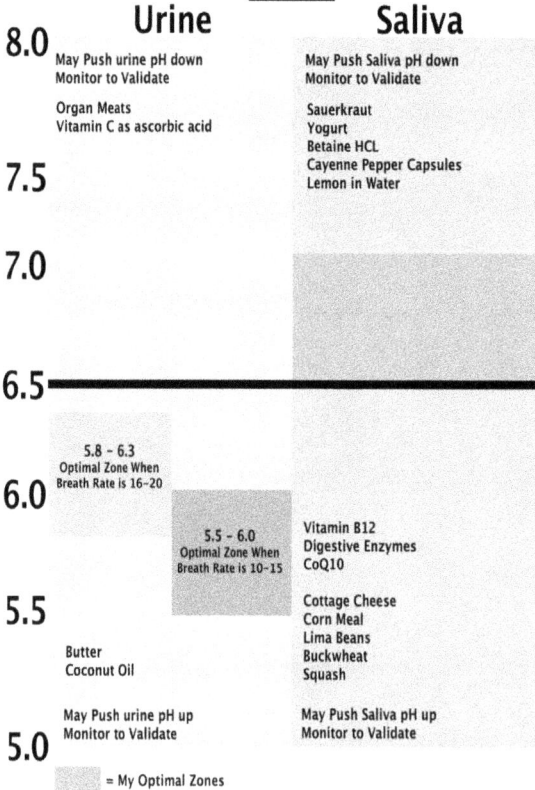

Energy Validators

Fat Burner	Carb Burner
__ Breath Rate < 15bpm	Breath Rate > 16bpm __
__ Breath Hold > 50sec	Breath Hold < 50sec __
__ Systolic BP > 133	Systolic BP < 112 __
__ Glucose > 100	Glucose < 70 __
__ Urine pH < 6.1	Urine pH > 6.3 __
__ Saliva pH > 6.9	Saliva pH < 6.6 __
__ Type II Diabetes	Irritable When Hungry __

Digestive Issue Validators

__ Systolic Blood Pressure < 112
__ Diastolic Blood Pressure < 74
__ Burping and/or Bloating
__ Passing Gas
__ Reflux/Heartburn
__ Light Colored Stool
__ Constipation
__ Urgent Diarrhea
__ Nausea

Needs Improvement

Electrolyte Deficiency Electrolyte Excess	Anabolic Catabolic	Carb Burner Fat Burner	Digestive Issues

Sample Completed *Imbalance Guide*

IMBALANCE GUIDE

Name: **Suzy Q**   Date: **Jan 4**   Time: **11:00 AM**

Electrolyte State

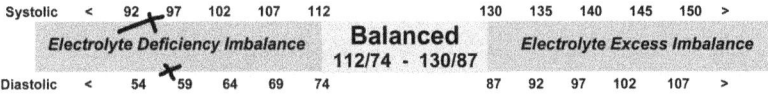

Systolic	<	92	97	102	107	112		130	135	140	145	150	>

Electrolyte Deficiency Imbalance **Balanced** 112/74 - 130/87 *Electrolyte Excess Imbalance*

Diastolic	<	54	59	64	69	74		87	92	97	102	107	>

Circle Your Breath Rate

Less Than 10
See Appendix C

10 (11) 12 13 14 15 16 17 18 19 20

More Than 20
See Appendix C

Breath Hold Time = 55 Seconds

pH Chart

Urine

8.0
May Push urine pH down
Monitor to Validate

Organ Meats
Vitamin C as ascorbic acid

7.5

7.0

6.5 ✗

5.8 – 6.3
Optimal Zone When
Breath Rate is 16–20

6.0

5.5 – 6.0
Optimal Zone When
Breath Rate is 10-15

5.5
Butter
Coconut Oil

May Push urine pH up
Monitor to Validate

5.0

= My Optimal Zones

Saliva

May Push Saliva pH down
Monitor to Validate

Sauerkraut
Yogurt
Betaine HCL
Cayenne Pepper Capsules
Lemon in Water

✗ (at 7.0)

Vitamin B12
Digestive Enzymes
CoQ10

Cottage Cheese
Corn Meal
Lima Beans
Buckwheat
Squash

May Push Saliva pH up
Monitor to Validate

Catabolic/Anabolic Validators

Catabolic	Anabolic
Urine pH < 6.1	Urine pH > 6.3 ✗
Saliva pH > 6.9	Saliva pH < 6.6
Oliguria	Polyuria
Soft/Loose Stool	Hard Stool / Constipation ✗
Wake Easily	Difficult to Rise
High Debris in Urine	Low Debris in Urine
Migraines	Anxiety

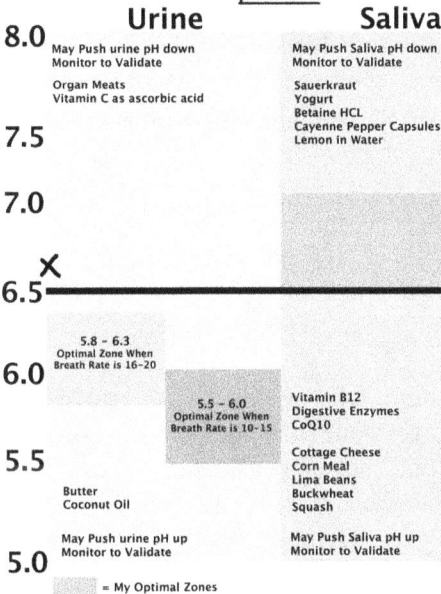

Energy Validators

Fat Burner	Carb Burner
✗ Breath Rate < 15bpm	Breath Rate > 16bpm
✗ Breath Hold > 50sec	Breath Hold < 50sec
Systolic BP > 133	Systolic BP < 112 ✗
Glucose > 100	Glucose < 70
Urine pH < 6.1	Urine pH > 6.3 ✗
Saliva pH > 6.9	Saliva pH < 6.6
Type II Diabetes	Irritable When Hungry

Digestive Issue Validators

✗ Systolic Blood Pressure < 112
✗ Diastolic Blood Pressure < 74
✗ Burping and/or Bloating
✗ Passing Gas
__ Reflux/Heartburn
__ Light Colored Stool
✗ Constipation
__ Urgent Diarrhea
__ Nausea

Needs Improvement

(Electrolyte Deficiency)   Anabolic   Carb Burner   (Digestive Issues)
Electrolyte Excess   Catabolic   Fat Burner

You should already have numbers on your *Data Tracking Sheet* from your self-tests. If you don't, what's the holdup? Are you trying to hurt me? Simply take the numbers from your *Data Tracking Sheet* and fill in your *Imbalance Guide*. Here is the easy breakdown:

Electrolyte State

On the red and green electrolyte state bar, according to your blood pressure reading, mark an "X" on the top of the bar, and another "X" on the bottom. The top "X" coincides with your systolic (top) blood pressure reading. The bottom "X" coincides with your diastolic (bottom) blood pressure reading. (Remember that "top" and "bottom" refer to systolic and diastolic, respectively. Yet, on most automatic blood pressure cuffs the very bottom number is your pulse.)

This section indicates if your electrolyte state is balanced, electrolyte deficient or electrolyte excess. The green zone is an optimal blood pressure reading of 112/74 to 130/90. If both of your "X" marks fall in the red zone on the left, that could indicate an Electrolyte Deficiency Imbalance. If both of your "X" marks fall in the red zone on the right, this could indicate an Electrolyte Excess Imbalance. In either case, the distance from the balanced green zone counts. If your systolic blood pressure is 165, that is quite a bit higher than 130 and a person may consider this an area that could use a lot of attention.

If only the top number or the bottom number pushes into the left or right red zones, you may be experiencing only a slight imbalance in that direction. For example, if your systolic pressure is 105, but your diastolic is 78, there may be only a slight Electrolyte Deficiency Imbalance.

Special note: If your systolic reading falls within the Electrolyte Deficiency Imbalance box on the left, yet your diastolic blood pressure (bottom number) is above 89, you would not be considered electrolyte deficient. However, if your diastolic blood pressure is over 90 on a regular basis, it may be time to have your doctor or health practitioner check that out.

A Word On Medications

If your systolic blood pressure is in the green zone, yet you are currently taking blood pressure lowering medications, you're really not that balanced at all, are you? If your doctor felt like you needed to be on blood pressure meds, odds are pretty great that you are experiencing an Electrolyte Excess Imbalance.

The same thing goes for the other direction. If you show a balanced blood pressure number, yet you're currently taking antidepressants, you may be dealing with an Electrolyte Deficiency Imbalance since depression medications can often restrict a person's ability to pee out salts, thereby raising blood pressure, in most cases.

Breath Rate and Breath Hold Time

Circle the number that corresponds with your breaths per minute (remember, you are counting only inhales, not inhales and exhales). You will use this information to determine your optimal urine pH zone. If your breath rate is below 10 or above 20, that's a problem. You may not need to call 911, but you do need to read *pH Balance – Acid/Alkaline Imbalances* in Appendix C. Taking steps to improve an abnormal breath rate can bring about a great deal of relief to someone who has been suffering for a long time.

Next to Breath Hold Time, simply fill in the number of seconds you were able to comfortably hold your breath.

Catabolic/Anabolic State

On your *Imbalance Guide*, notice the heading, pH Chart. For both urine and saliva you see optimal green zones. This is where most people want their pHs to fall. There are two different green zones for urine that overlap because the optimal zone for urine pH changes according to your breath rate. In this regard, if your breath rate changes due to nutritional changes you make, be sure to shoot for the optimal green zone according to your breath rate. *The Coalition* has an amazing tool called a pH Balancing Chart that changes the green zones for you automatically. I teach you how to use that later in this chapter.

Look at the urine and saliva pH numbers that you recorded on your *Data Tracking Sheet* and place an "X" for each of those numbers onto the pH Chart. If either of your pHs fall outside of those optimal zones, you may want give this area some attention. If your pHs fall within both green zones, you may be balanced in this area. It's okay to be balanced; that is what you're shooting for.

You also see foods or supplements listed in each quadrant of the pH chart. The top left quadrant lists foods or supplements that may help push urine pH down. The bottom left are items that can help push urine pH up. The same idea occurs on the right side for saliva. With these guides, you can see which foods or supplements may help push you closer to a balanced state.

Under Catabolic/Anabolic Validators on your *Imbalance Guide*, below each heading you see a box that represents sample pH readings that are common for each imbalance. With an Anabolic Imbalance, urine pH is commonly higher and closer to the saliva pH reading. With a Catabolic Imbalance, the urine pH is commonly lower and further away from the saliva reading. In other words, in a Catabolic Imbalance, there is more distance between the urine and saliva pH numbers.

Below these sample readings are common symptoms that can accompany each imbalance. Check off any that frequently apply to you. Again, don't assume you have an imbalance just because you experience the symptoms. Use the symptoms only as validation of numbers that are indicating a possible imbalance.

Special Notes

Under "Catabolic," oliguria means that you do not urinate frequently, or maybe you urinate frequently, but in small amounts. Under "Anabolic," polyuria means you urinate frequently, with volume.
High or low debris in urine is asking, if you pee in a cup, do you see a lot of debris floating around in your urine?
On the catabolic side, only check off "Migraines" if your headaches frequently originate in the back of your head or neck. If you get frontal headaches, those are not generally migraines and you should not check this box.

Energy Production

Under Energy Validators, check off the points that are appropriate for you, whether they be numbers from your self-tests or symptoms you experience. If you were unable to run some of the numbers, like glucose, leave that space blank and simply use the data that you do have.

If one side shows a predominant number of checks, you may be experiencing that imbalance. If checks are distributed fairly evenly between both sides, then you are likely balanced in your energy production and that is a good thing. Concern yourself with one of these imbalances only if you appear to sway strongly in one direction. For example, if you have five or six items checked on one side and maybe only one or two on the other.

<u>Digestive Issues</u>

If you can check off any of the items listed under Digestive Issues, it would be wise to focus on improving digestion.

Conclusions

Finally, draw some type of conclusion. Any conclusions you find may change as you make adjustments to your nutrition, however, the idea is to come to a conclusion. Are you balanced in all areas? Do you need a lot of attention in the area of electrolytes but everything else looks good? Where are you? Come to a conclusion so you will know which imbalances to pay attention to while I explain them in the next chapter.

Under the Needs Improvement section, select any imbalances that you feel could use help. If you feel that the imbalance is strong (or severe) and needs a lot of work, you can circle that imbalance. If you feel that the imbalance is present, but could maybe just use a little attention, you can underline that imbalance. Keep this *Imbalance Guide* handy while you read through the rest of the book so you can remember which imbalances need attention. This will be helpful as I go over foods and supplement choices that can be used to improve specific imbalances.

Keep in mind that the tools I have provided for you to get a glimpse of your chemistry will give you just that: A glimpse. I have placed intermediate testing procedures in Appendix B and people can learn even more in-depth information about their own body by working with a professional health coach. When looking at only a few biological markers, imbalances can be disguised or misinterpreted. With this in mind, I suggest only taking major steps to push an imbalance in the optimal direction if that imbalance appears to be strong. After all, the goal should be to become balanced, not to create another imbalance in the opposite direction.

In chapter nine I explain how these imbalances can affect your health, your life and your weight.

Wha'd He Say?

In this chapter, you learned:

- Interpreting your numbers on your *Imbalance Guide* is the first step toward understanding why other diets have failed you in the past.
- When deciding if you are dealing with a specific imbalance or not, the measurements are your greatest influence. Symptoms should be used only as a confirmation marker. Do not mark yourself as having an imbalance simply because you are experiencing symptoms often seen with that imbalance.
- If you appear to be experiencing a strong imbalance on your *Imbalance Guide*, go to the bottom of the page and circle that imbalance. If you appear to have a slight imbalance, you can underline that imbalance at the bottom of the *Imbalance Guide*. If you appear to be balanced in that area, don't mark that imbalance at all.
- If you understand which imbalances may be giving you trouble, you will now know which information to pay more attention to for the rest of the book.

CHAPTER NINE

How Imbalances Cause Weight Gain

This information will be your secret weapon. Beyond improving digestion, many readers won't have a lot of imbalances that need improving. But if imbalances show up on your *Imbalance Guide,* you may finally be able to move past those hurdles that have been sabotaging diet after diet. Time to jump into how these imbalances can sabotage weight loss efforts left and right.

Electrolyte State

The electrolyte state is defined by blood pressure (though a professional health coach may have equipment that can look at other variables in this equation, like conductivity of urine and saliva).

In the world of natural health, where the terrain of the body gives so many insights into how the body is functioning, if an imbalance can exist in one direction, there must be an opposite to that imbalance. Otherwise, there would be no middle ground, no place where the body could be considered "balanced." Seems reasonable, right? By the time you finish this book, you will likely realize how ridiculous it is that the medical world puts so much attention on high blood pressure, but totally ignores an equally debilitating imbalance in the other direction.

Imbalance - Electrolyte Deficiency

When blood pressure is low, this is often a reflection of low mineral content in the bloodstream. When the mineral levels decrease, it is a reflection of a decrease in your salts or the vascular system being too

113

open (dilated). Our mineral content not only comes from actual salt, but from our food too. As I covered in chapter three, if your digestion is not working properly, you can't assimilate the minerals from the food you're eating and the mineral content in the system can decrease. There are a few other contributing factors that could possibly result in low blood pressure and I will get back to this soon.

Very few doctors will ever talk to you about your blood pressure being low. Since there is no drug for low blood pressure, the ramifications are not in their training. We all know that high blood pressure can cause heart attacks and strokes (blowouts). When they say your blood pressure is great even though it's too low, they're saying that you'll never have a blowout. But is it fun to run around on flat tires all day? An optimal blood pressure reading is said to be 120 over 80. So, if 140 over 90 is considered high blood pressure in the medical world, wouldn't having those numbers off by the same amount in the other direction be regarded as low blood pressure? Shouldn't a reading of 100 over 70 be considered low?

The minerals, or salts, in the system represent the conductivity, or ability for electricity to flow through the system. When the mineral content is low, there's no spark; and energy can be low. Without this energy, the brain can't function at its full potential, a result created by the lack of minerals required for signals to travel through. Many people with depression, and even other manifestations of "mental illness," are often just cases where there is not enough mineral in the system. Low mineral levels often mean there's not enough spark to give the brain what it needs to function correctly, or there is not enough mineral to control blood pH sufficiently. Of course, blood sugar is a big player in this regard also, but I get into that in a bit.

We seem to have the mindset that, if what we're eating is providing us with enough energy to stand up and walk to our car, we have all the resources we need. But every task that our bodies handle needs resources to complete it. Vitamins, minerals, amino acids—they're all important. The mineral in the system is very important because, without it, there is no way for signals to travel from the body to the brain. It's like electricity in water. If you put an electrical current in water, you get shocked and it's really not that fun. You get shocked because that water contains minerals; and that current can travel through the minerals. But if you put a current in distilled water, with no mineral in it, the current doesn't travel. It's the same way with the human brain. If signals can't travel, the brain doesn't work optimally and we feel depressed, tired or lethargic or, in the worst cases, maybe we think that we're a fire truck. Almost all of the clients with depression issues who have come to me, or to any of my colleagues, have shown a low blood pressure reading (unless they are taking an antidepressant that is raising their blood pressure artificially). There are exceptions to every rule. I mean just the other day I saw a guy with a mullet that actually looked good, so there can be a first time for everything. But generally speaking, the majority of clients I see with depression symptoms have low blood pressure.

The brain needs fuel just like anything else. If your toaster isn't working, what's the first thing you check? You look to see if it's plugged in. You don't send your toaster to therapy or soak it in medication; you just look to see if it's getting the juice it needs to function properly. I'm not saying that therapy can't be beneficial for some people; I'm just saying that, when it comes to mechanical objects, we have the sense to look at a malfunction and try to figure out what is causing that object to function at a substandard level. However, when it comes to people, we don't check to see if they have the resources for their "machine" to perform optimally. We just assume they must have daddy abandonment issues, or felt inadequate as a child because their brother was always the first one to find the prize in the bottom of the cereal box. Yes, it can be very upsetting to think back on the terror of your brother having fun with all the press-on tattoos while you had none; but if your brain had the resources to function at its full potential, it would be easier to look past that and move on with your life, now that you're 36.

Don't feel like I'm downplaying depression issues just because I'm talking like a jerk. I've experienced these issues first-hand and they can be very troubling, confusing, and a huge pile of not-at-all-fun. They were especially confusing for me because I had always been a very positive person; then all of a sudden, I just wanted to ball up on the floor and cry at old episodes of *The Brady Bunch*. Once I understood how these issues can come out of nowhere, what imbalances most often create them and how to improve those imbalances, I was right back to my old self and could once again laugh at the fact that it *was* Mom's favorite vase and she *did* always say don't play ball in the house. (Non-Brady fans will have no idea what I'm talking about here and may think I'm a little drunk right now.) You can learn more about why this happens and how to improve these issues in my upcoming book, *Done With Depression.* But for now, I simply want to lay down a foundation that can help you understand how the body needs nourishment to do all the things it does. The body can't just show up to work every day and make it all magically happen. Resources are needed to keep your "machine" running properly.

In chapter six I explained how a lack of minerals can create cravings. If an Electrolyte Deficiency Imbalance shows up in your numbers, you will certainly want to take steps to correct it so you can get those cravings under control. Once your body learns that junk food can thicken the blood to raise blood pressure AND trigger pleasure sensors in the brain that trick the body into thinking resources are on the way, this can be a person's only way out of depression. Any wonder why people might continue to eat junk all the time if they were dealing with an Electrolyte Deficiency Imbalance? The good news is, this can be corrected.

Since sugar (or glucose) is a factor when measuring blood pressure, understand what can happen if you begin to reduce the number of sugars, carbs or starches you are consuming. As glucose levels come down, blood pressure will come down as well, unless you have implemented methods to raise your mineral levels. This is why, if you are experiencing an Electrolyte Deficiency Imbalance, it is so important to raise mineral levels if you want to reduce your carb intake.

Imbalance - Electrolyte Excess

If an Electrolyte Deficiency Imbalance normally indicates a lack of electrolytes, the opposite would be a state where too many electrolytes are present. This is called an Electrolyte Excess Imbalance.

In general, high blood pressure can be an expression of insufficient, or lousy, kidney function. This means that, when excessive electrolytes become concentrated in the bodily fluids, it's usually a result of insufficient hydration (not drinking enough clean water) or impaired excretion of mineral salts through the kidneys. High blood pressure can also result from a constricted vascular system. In any case, electrolyte stress can lead to hypertension (high blood pressure) and other circulatory and cardiovascular problems. A vascular system that is constricted often points to an autonomic nervous system issue or a buildup on the arterial walls. (I talk more about the autonomic nervous system when I talk about Sympathetic and Parasympathetic Imbalances in Appendix C if you're interested.)

If kidneys are not working optimally, or a person is not drinking enough water to wash the junk out, excess filth will accumulate. You learned in chapter two that excess filth can be stored in fat cells if the body is too overwhelmed to remove that junk. Therefore, improving this imbalance can result in a cleaner, lighter you. If your *Imbalance Guide* showed an Electrolyte Excess Imbalance, have you gotten up to go get a glass of water yet? Go!

Catabolic/Anabolic States

At the cellular level, the body is always in an anabolic or catabolic state, or in the process of switching back and forth between the two. During the day, our cell membranes are intended to open up (much like a flower) so nutrients can get in and out more easily. This "more open" state is called a catabolic state. At night, our cell membranes are intended to become more closed (again, like a flower) so nutrients cannot get in and out as easily. This "more closed" state is called an anabolic state. Both states are appropriate, and even necessary, for a body to function optimally. Due to many possible factors, some people can get stuck in one state and their body will not switch back and forth as intended.

To make the body operate correctly, we need to oscillate back and forth from the anabolic state at night, while we sleep and rebuild, and a catabolic state during the day, while we're active. Without this natural oscillation, many problems can occur. Let's go over each of these imbalances individually and cover how each one can lead to weight gain in its own right. You okay with that?

Imbalance - Anabolic

First of all, there are many benefits that take place while a body is in an anabolic state. This is the state where the body engages in most of its repairing or rebuilding processes. You've probably heard the word anabolic in reference to steroids. Weightlifters take anabolic steroids in order to be in the tissue building, anabolic state when they are not playing fair with muscle building. If a guy begins to add some muscle, he may think, "This is nice, but I'd really like to be so big that my neck completely disappears and I can no longer hold my arms down at my sides. I want my arms to always look like they are sticking straight out like Ralphie's little brother, Randy, from *A Christmas Story* when he was wearing his winter parka. That's what I want to look like." By using these anabolic steroids, this guy can keep his body in an anabolic, muscle-building state most of the time.

While an anabolic state can have its benefits, any state can cause problems when pushed to an extreme—even problems beyond becoming so huge that you look more like a video game character than a human. Although it is very appropriate for the cells to be in an anabolic state at night, some individuals will stay in a more anabolic state most of the time. These individuals are said to be experiencing an Anabolic Imbalance.

This Anabolic Imbalance can also cause constipation by sending too much of the body's water to the kidneys and not enough to the bowels, making the stool harder and more difficult to move. An Anabolic Imbalance can also cause individuals to pee high volumes of urine frequently throughout the day. They will often have to get up in the middle of the night to tinkle.

In this anabolic state, an individual can have a hard time dropping weight for a number of reasons. If a person is constipated, they aren't removing junk the way the body is intended to. We don't poop to support the toilet paper industry. We poop to remove junk.

Beyond the possible constipation issues, if people are stuck in the anabolic state most of the time, they can hold on to too much stuff at the cellular level. The catabolic state is where tissues break down and the body gets rid of junk. If a person never moves into the catabolic state, that trash removal part of the day isn't happening and this person will have a very hard time dropping weight.

Imbalance - Catabolic

The catabolic state is where the body kind of "breaks down and cleans house," so to speak. In a catabolic state, the body is primed to use oxygen to create energy, so it is appropriate to be in a catabolic state during your waking hours to keep you going all day. This, along with what I just explained about the anabolic state, helps to show how both the anabolic and catabolic states are appropriate during the appropriate times. However, in the same way that I talked about people who lean too anabolic, some individuals will stay in a more catabolic state most of the time. These individuals are said to be experiencing a Catabolic Imbalance.

If someone is stuck in a catabolic state, the cell walls are too permeable and this individual will often burn up muscle and protein and even membrane fats. Breaking down tissues and muscle so they can be rebuilt is a beneficial aspect of the catabolic state, but when a person is in that state too often, for too long, that "cleaning house" process can turn into a body that is flat out falling apart. If you bulldoze your garage to add a new wing to your house, your house could increase its value. But if you knock down your garage just because you're addicted to knocking things down, your neighbors won't like you, just like you won't like your body if you're unable to move back into that "rebuilding" state. The more muscle we lose, the lower our metabolism, and we may burn less fat. A Catabolic Imbalance can also make the bile too thick and sticky to flow properly, therefore restricting digestion and restricting the body's ability to remove junk. That's not good.

Insomnia is very common with a Catabolic Imbalance because the cell membranes are more permeable, which is a characteristic of the daytime state. These people can't sleep because their bodies are still awake and operating at full speed. Most sleeping aids will knock you out in the head so you can sleep, but your body will still be wide awake all night. As a result, you might either wake up exhausted or you become tired again a few hours after waking. I guess it depends on your candle, and how short it has become by burning both ends at once. The point is, I'd like to teach you how to fix the problem instead of just selling you more candles.

In relation to weight gain, it is very common for a catabolic person to be insulin resistant. You will remember from chapter five that when insulin levels are high, your body can't burn stored fat for fuel; and, even worse, the high insulin sends the signal to store more fat to be used as fuel later. This can be a common cause for weight gain in overly catabolic individuals. With insulin resistance, the body may need to produce two or three times the amount of insulin to handle normal amounts of glucose. For example, let's say that when the average person eats a turkey sandwich, insulin production is at "level six" on a scale of one to ten. But if an individual is insulin resistant, that person may need to produce insulin at a level of twelve, or even fifteen, to handle the same amount of glucose that others could take care of with much less insulin.

This greater amount of insulin not only causes the body to store more fat and blocks the body from burning stored fat for even longer, it also slams the cells with a much greater load of insulin. Like any drug or hormone, the cells will eventually stop listening (or responding) and one can become insulin resistant. That's what Type II Diabetes is all about. The cells are no longer responding to the insulin, and sugar accumulates in the bloodstream.

Energy Production

The next two imbalances I cover are Fat Burner Imbalance and Carb Burner Imbalance. These deal with energy production and how the body uses food for fuel. Before I explain energy production, understand that I will be leaving out complicated methods the body can use to create energy. They are not important for this explanation.

To create energy, simply speaking, our bodies burn either fat or glucose. Your body is designed to burn both types of fuel for different purposes. Despite that, changes can occur in our bodies, or in our lives, that will train our bodies to prefer one fuel over the other. The body may stop burning the other type of fuel almost entirely. This is another reason why there is no such thing as the diet that is right for everyone. It doesn't exist. Some people burn fats much better than glucose and some people are the opposite. This really puts all these arguments into perspective about "low-carb," "low-fat," "high-protein," "the drunk diet," "I only eat things that start with the letter F..." I could go on for days. They're still all going to be wrong. In order to find the right "diet," you really need to look at the person, because each person processes foods differently. Good thing you're looking at your own person right now by following the steps in this book.

Remember, I've greatly simplified the two imbalances below. My main concern is that you understand a body can prefer to burn one type of fuel over the other and this can affect the types of foods that may be optimal for that person to consume.

Imbalance - Carb Burner

Carb Burners are people who are predisposed to burn off all their glucose and do not seem to burn fat very well. Now, it's not that they won't burn fat, but they will always prefer to burn off all their glucose first. If the body prefers not to burn stored fat, a person can have a hard time losing weight.

Imbalance - Fat Burner

If you find that you show indications of having a Fat Burner Imbalance, you most likely are burning much more fat than glucose. If you also have high cholesterol, high triglycerides and a high fasting glucose, any of these markers can be another indication that you are not processing glucose effectively.

Many individuals who are overweight and have this imbalance will ask, "How is it that I'm burning mostly fat but I'm still so fat?" This is because their bodies are turning almost every carb and sugar that they eat into fat. In order to process sugar or glucose, the body is having to take all sugar or glucose coming in and turn it into fat before it is able to be "burned" for energy.

Using The Coalition

In chapter seven I introduced you to *The Coalition for Health Education*, which can be found at www.OurCoalition.org. I recommend joining to all those who plan on monitoring their own chemistry. The tools provided to members on *The Coalition* website are by far the best tracking and monitoring tools of their kind available to consumers. If you plan to use the guidelines presented in this book without monitoring your own chemistry, you're just a silly, silly person. Without watching what your numbers do, how are you going to know when to adjust the things you are implementing to balance your body? How are you going to know if you're making progress and how are you going to know when it's time to slow your efforts so you don't create an imbalance in the other direction? You have to monitor. You have to be a participant in your own health. A monitoring device is not something you own and ignore like the treadmill you hang your clothes on. A monitoring device is something you actively use. The days of allowing someone to tell you,

"Take these pills and come back to see me in two months" are over. You wouldn't be reading this book if you found that route worked for you. The sooner you come to the realization that you're going to have to put forth some effort, the sooner you'll improve your current circumstances and reap the rewards that come with responsible ownership of your own mechanism (by mechanism, I mean you).

Once you have an indication of what imbalances are giving you the most trouble, you can log in to your account on *The Coalition* and begin learning more about those imbalances and different ways to improve them. You can start to input your weekly self-test numbers into the progress charts to get a visual of how your numbers are moving and the progress you're making. There is even a graph for your "well-being" so you can monitor how the way you feel changes according to where your chemistry is. As you learn where your body seems to function optimally, you can start to get an idea of how to keep your chemistry in the place where you feel the best. Is that like cheating or what? I just love how sneaky that is, to look inside your own body and know exactly what is needed to feel your best. Who knew we would ever be able to do that?

The Coalition also provides you with a food journal system like no other. For each day, you can input what you're eating, how you're feeling, any symptoms that have come up or improved, etc. Then, when you enter self-test results in your progress charts, those results also show up in your food journal next to the appropriate time. Now, you can look at the foods you eat and see how those foods affect your chemistry and how you feel later that day. This can really help you pinpoint the foods and choices that are working best for you. No more throwing darts blindly at the menu of life. This can give you a clear-cut visual of the optimal diet for you... and you're in charge of the menu.

The jewel of *The Coalition* is the pH Balancing Chart. This is some good stuff. As I described in chapter eight, your urine pH has an optimal zone that changes according to your breath rate. If your breath rate is above sixteen, you will normally do well with a urine pH between 5.8 and 6.3 and a saliva pH between 6.5 and 7.0. If your breath rate is below 16, you will normally do well with a urine pH between 5.5 and 6.0 and a saliva pH between 6.5 and 7.0.

The pH Balancing Chart on *The Coalition* maps all that for you. Once you enter at least one urine pH entry and one saliva pH entry and one breath rate and breath hold entry, the system will create your pH balancing chart and display it within your personalized site. This chart will show you your optimal pH zones for both urine and saliva, and bring in your most recent pH entries from your progress charts so you can see if you're in your optimal zones or not. If you're out of your optimal zones, the chart lists foods and supplements that can help push those pHs in the right direction. It's an amazing tool and worth ten times the price of admission all by itself. Since I assisted *The Coalition* in creating this particular gadget, if it helps you improve your health as much as I believe it will, I think you should show your appreciation by sending me a new pair of flip-flops. I have a really hard time picking out flip-flops, but when they come to me as a gift I always seem to enjoy them.

Improving Imbalances

Throughout the rest of the book I provide you with ways to improve all six of these imbalances. Be patient, these imbalances were not created in a week and you will not likely correct them in a week. However, for some issues that come with these imbalances, I will be able to teach you methods that could bring improvement quickly.

Wha'd He Say?

In this chapter, you learned:

- Don't forget about digestive issues. If you're a person who has a hard time losing weight or sticking to a diet, some type of digestive issue is very often at play.
- You MUST monitor your progress. If you don't monitor while trying to improve an imbalance, you won't know when it's time to reduce your efforts, and you may create an imbalance in the other direction. Just because your imbalance may have lead to weight gain, that does not mean the opposite side of that imbalance will lead to weight loss. Both sides can cause weight gain, but for different reasons. Balance is the key.

CHAPTER TEN

Fat is Not Making You Fat

Fat Does Not Come From Fat

Most avid dieters understand this principle by now and, for you, this will not be groundbreaking information. But for those of you who are still living in the eighties, when every nutrition expert told us to cut the fat, I want to cover this here. Please step away from your arcade-size Ms. Pacman and prepare to be enlightened.

Your body fat is not merely a result of fat that you consumed. This has been common knowledge for so long now, and yet I still have clients tell me all time, "I made sure I only ate low-fat stuff." If the label says "low-fat," it usually means that product will make you fat. When manufacturers take fats out of food, they often replace those fats with chemicals, sugars and artificial sweeteners to give it flavor. These replacements cause the body to store fat more than most fats do.

There are fats that are not healthy, like trans fats and that stuff that drips off the french fry cage of the deep fryer. However, our bodies require nutritional fats in order to function properly. By consuming fats appropriate for your body, you can actually accelerate weight loss. There are bodily processes that could not be completed without fats. If you're not consuming enough healthy fats in your diet, your body will hold on to stored fat like it's money in the bank.

Believing a low-fat diet is the best weight loss plan is a thing of the past. Now that we understand the science behind consuming fats, we realize that entire low-fat train of thought was a huge screw-up. Just remember how easy it was for our culture to believe this myth for nearly a decade. When false information spreads through the public for so long, it can take quite some time for the truth to reach everyone, if it ever does. This understanding may make it easier for you to believe some of the other common mistakes being made in the world of nutrition, and elsewhere.

"A lie gets halfway around the world before the truth has a chance to get its pants on."
                                                    - Winston Churchill

The Saturated Fat Conspiracy

This might bug you a lot. Not because I'm going to tell you something else that you shouldn't eat, but because you may come to the conclusion that you've been avoiding great foods in the name of bad science. Long ago, a bunch of scientists discovered a correlation between high levels of saturated fats (particularly a type of saturated fat called palmitic acid) and cardiovascular disease. They concluded that, because so many heart attack victims had high levels of these saturated fats, we should avoid consuming saturated fats. Due to the fact that egg yolks and red meat both contain higher levels of saturated fats, these foods became the red-headed stepchild of the nutrition world.

Newsflash: Those high levels of the saturated fat palmitic acid don't come from consuming saturated fats. Here's how it works: The body stores glucose from carbohydrates in the liver and muscle tissues in the form of glycogen. Once these stores are full, many excess sugars get converted into palmitic acid and stored as a saturated fat. This is the cause of elevated levels of saturated fats for most of those suffering from cardiovascular disease. It's excess carb and sugar consumption; consuming saturated fats has little to do with that equation at all. These fats can also group with glycerol to form triglycerides. High triglyceride levels are said to be a common risk factor for cardiovascular disease.

Cholesterol

The same misguided thinking that had us shy away from saturated fats also had us running in horror from cholesterol. It's time you knew the truth. Approximately 85% of our cholesterol stores are made by our liver. Only about 15% comes from our diet. Since cholesterol has so many important functions, when we decrease our dietary intake of cholesterol to lower our cholesterol numbers, our bodies just makes more cholesterol to make up for the deficit. Cholesterol is used to repair damage done by high amounts of insulin in the bloodstream, so it would make sense that when insulin goes high, cholesterol would go high too. To lower your cholesterol, lower your carbohydrate and sugar intake, or whatever is causing too much free radical activity—not your cholesterol intake.

Genetics can play a role in how the body is predisposed to operate, but we can normally control the outcome with nutrition and lifestyle changes. Usually a whole family will have high cholesterol because they all grew up eating in a similar fashion, not necessarily because it is in their genes.

There is rarely a malfunction in the body that makes one person make more cholesterol than another for no reason. Your body is making a high amount of cholesterol to fix a problem. With a high portion of the American public being predisposed to insulin resistance, the problem, most commonly, is that the insulin levels are too high. Your body makes more cholesterol to patch up the damage that the high insulin is causing. Yes, as the body patches up more and more damage, the passages can get smaller and smaller and eventually clog up with "excess cholesterol." However, blaming the problem on the cholesterol would be like blaming firemen for fires... "Well, every time I see a fire there are all these guys in yellow jackets and red trucks all over the place. If we get rid of them, there would be no more fires." Why not just lower the insulin levels so your body won't need to make so much cholesterol? Hmmm.

For decades the medical world told us that 220 was the optimal number for total cholesterol in the bloodstream. A few years ago, the medical world came out with "new findings" stating that our cholesterol truly should be below 200. Well, let's say that 35% of the population has a total cholesterol number that falls between 200 - 220. The range that was considered to be healthy for decades. What happens to that 35% of the population when medical authorities lower the suggested blood cholesterol range to below 200? That 35% all become prescription buying customers, that's what. Wouldn't that give the cholesterol medication manufacturers a 35% increase in sales overnight? Is that the most brilliant marketing you've ever heard? I don't even think Justin Bieber could top that.

126

Again, good, free-range eggs (including the yolk) and good meat can be excellent dietary choices. Don't be afraid of the saturated fat or the cholesterol, and don't let some Barney tell you otherwise.

Coconut Oil

Don't forget, it is my opinion that there is no food or supplement that is right for everyone when it comes to weight loss, or even improving health. But if anything could come close to fitting those criteria, coconut oil would be the winner.

Before I explain the benefits of coconut oil, let me first explain the circumstance in which coconut oil might not be a helpful tool for weight loss. If you fall into any of these categories, I suggest fixing the described issue so that you *can* use coconut oil.

1. If your bile is not flowing properly, it may be difficult for you to emulsify the fats in coconut oil and digest those fats correctly. If fats are not correctly processed, they can become a problem the body has to deal with. If enough undigested fats accumulate in the body, they can be stored as body fat or the body may attempt to push the fats out through the skin. This can create breakouts or make you the zit captain. If you need to improve your bile flow, use Beet Flow described in chapter three.
2. If a strong Anabolic Imbalance showed up on your *Imbalance Guide*, you may want to take steps toward improving that imbalance before you begin to use coconut oil. For some people, coconut oil can have a slight pro-anabolic effect so if you're already too anabolic, you don't want to use something that could push you more anabolic until you have introduced foods or supplements that can help correct that imbalance.
3. If you are constipated or have a hard stool, you may want to do the work to improve your constipation before introducing coconut oil. Moving a constipated person more anabolic can exacerbate constipation. But once you have corrected your Anabolic Imbalance or your constipation, you should be able to use coconut oil moderately and experience its amazing weight loss benefits.

But It Contains So Much Fat!

I know!!! That's the point. Coconut oil contains healthy fats that your body needs desperately to function properly. Coconut oil is one of the easiest ways to supply your body with those fats every day. Once your body starts to see these healthy fats coming into the system day after day, there won't be that need to be so stingy, holding on to all of your stored fat. If the body is receiving healthy fats every day, it feels better about burning off stored fat and you can lose weight.

As I explained in chapter two, I consume four to six tablespoons of coconut oil per day. That means I'm taking in up to seventy eight grams of saturated fat per day, just in coconut oil. That doesn't include any eggs, meats or other foods I eat. That doesn't mean that you need to consume that much, I have just found it to work well for me. Just be sure to use an extra virgin variety of coconut oil.

Here are some great ways to include coconut oil in your diet every day:

1. Cook with it - Many oils that are good for you, like extra virgin olive oil, have the ability to become toxic once the oil is heated. Coconut oil holds up to heat better than just about any other oil. At first, coconut oil may taste a little different with certain foods, like eggs. However, sooner or later your body will realize it can really utilize coconut oil, your taste buds will change, and you will end up enjoying it much more than any other oil. All that being said, cooking with it alone is usually not enough to get crazy weight loss results.

2. I add half to a full tablespoon of coconut oil to the skillet anytime I'm making a stir fry or eggs, etc. I have met people who don't like the smell of coconut oil once it has been cooked. For those individuals, Aunt Patty's brand makes a coconut oil that is odorless when cooked.

3. Add a tablespoon to a shake - When coconut oil gets cool, or even cold, it will harden. Therefore, if you don't have anything else of substance in your shake, like kale, it can get a little clumpy in the liquid when it gets cold. But if you use a good blender and add something else for the coconut oil to mix with, you won't really notice it and it will add a nice flavor.

4. Just eat it - Yes, just eat the coconut oil right out of the jar. I have a lot of clients who will eat a teaspoon of coconut oil after every

meal that they consume at home. It can be a little hard to carry coconut oil around in your pocket so if you only eat the oil while you're home, that's still better than none. Although... Artisana brand now makes organic raw coconut oil in little ketchup-sized packets. Just don't get the coconut butter because that contains more sugars. The packets of coconut oil contain a little over one ounce, which would equate to just over two tablespoons.

Keep in mind that coconut oil should always be consumed with a meal. You want that digestive action going on to help you properly emulsify the fats.

My Coconut Yummies recipe - This is the greatest trick ever for sneaking healthy fats into your diet and relieving the desire for something sweet after every meal. Below I share my recipe for a great after-dinner mint that can make you feel more satiated, dramatically aid weight loss and allow you to have a little treat at the end of each meal.

Coconut Yummies

Melt a cup of coconut oil in the oven or a toaster oven. You can also melt your coconut oil by placing the container in hot water in the sink. Either method can take a few minutes, but do not use a microwave just because it may be quicker! Next, I stir in half a packet of stevia and about 20-40 drops of flavored stevia. Optionally, you can open up four or five capsules of Pau D' Arco and mix them in too. Pau D' Arco is an herb commonly used for its anti-microbial properties, but it can add an almost chocolate-like taste to the coconut oil. As an alternative, you can add cinnamon or mint if you prefer those flavors.

To mold the coconut oil into little treats, I use silicone mini-muffin baking dishes. You can see the type I use under BOOK TOOLS > HELPFUL LINKS at www.DoneWithThatBooks.com.

I put about a tablespoon or a tablespoon and a half in each mini-muffin hole and put the batch in the fridge to harden.

Enjoy The Fats

Enjoying appropriate fats in your diet can make a world of difference to any weight loss effort, as long as you correct any digestive issues so you have the ability to process those fats. Most low-calorie diets eventually fail because they leave the person feeling hungry all the time. Fats can make you feel more satisfied and sustain energy longer. I go over more sources for good dietary fats in chapter fourteen. I even give you food options containing fats that can help to improve specific imbalances.

Wha'd He Say?

In this chapter, you learned:

- Consuming fat in your diet is not normally the cause of excess body fat.
- Our bodies require nutritional fats in order to function properly.
- Saturated fats are not evil.
- High cholesterol and high levels of saturated fats in the blood are normally caused by excessive sugar or carbohydrate consumption. Consuming cholesterol does not raise blood cholesterol levels over time.
- Coconut oil is an excellent tool to help the body drop stored fat. Coconut oil should be used only with proper bile flow. If you have an Anabolic Imbalance or chronic constipation issues, improve these problems before implementing coconut oil.

Chapter Eleven

Emotional Issues & The Psycho Factor

Avoiding The Psycho Factor

My upcoming books, *Done With Being Crazy*, *Done With Depression*, and *Done With Eating Disorders*, will all cover the many aspects of trouble that can be exacerbated by the "burn more calories than you consume" weight loss plan.

In chapter nine, under *Electrolyte Deficiency Imbalance*, I talked about mental and emotional problems that can develop from the body dealing with a lack of resources. You'll remember my talking about how, when your toaster doesn't work, you first look to see if it's plugged in. Many issues that people consider strictly psychological are frequently circumstances where the brain is not getting the fuel it needs to function correctly. If physiological circumstances or poor lifestyle choices are restricting the amount of fuel that could make it to a person's brain, what do you think is going to happen when this poor guy tries to create a caloric deficit in order to lose some weight? Yes, you guessed it... The Psycho Factor kicks in.

Promise me you won't dig into your four-year psychology degree and write me letters explaining that some girls have eating disorders because they were traumatized by their Uncle Biff who locked them in a closet and forced them to eat a case of Twinkies. I know people deal with legitimate issues in their lives and I go over that later in this chapter. However, you'll also remember that, in chapter six, I explained how these same people who are dealing with an issue they consider to be a ten, on a scale of one to ten, can bring that down to a three or four, once the brain is getting the fuel it needs to function optimally. So, even though the problem may have other underlying circumstances attached, in most cases, these problems become a lot easier to deal with when the person is working with a brain that is receiving optimal resources. Most problems have more than one cause. In this book, I'm looking at the biological or physiological issues. Often times, lifting these burdens can make the emotional side easier to work with.

Some of these issues can be a lot more complicated than what I'm explaining here, and will be dissected further in the titles I mentioned at the beginning of the chapter. I bring this up here only to further explain how creating a calorie deficit is not the optimal idea that many present. I use these points also to emphasize how using more medium-carb meals can help you avoid any Psycho Factor moments if you see them creeping in due to a decrease in your carb or sugar consumption.

It's pretty common for people to go a little crazy while they're trying to lose weight. A popular candy bar ad campaign that runs constantly on television right now is all about how people turn into someone else when they're hungry. This chapter is about learning how to avoid those moments of insanity, no matter how little or big your crazy fits can sometimes be. The point is: There is no point in losing weight if the diet you're using makes you miserable or emotionally unstable. How are you going to sustain that in a manner that will allow you to keep the weight off? The trick is to lose weight while you're making sure your brain gets all the fuel it needs.

Why Do Pregnant Women Gain Fat And Go Nuts?

I like to use the weight gain that can accompany pregnancy as an example because it's such an extreme situation. It clearly illustrates how a lack of resources can not only lead to weight gain, it can also lead to those moments of "unreasonableness," a.k.a. The Psycho Factor. It doesn't matter how sweet, caring, generous or mentally stable a woman is, at some point while she's pregnant, we all know she's going to snap and we all know none of us will hold it against her. It's common knowledge and we all accept it. Now you're going to get to understand why it happens.

To make a baby takes a lot of minerals and other types of nutrients. Believe it or not, babies aren't just delivered by a stork; it takes resources to build a baby just like it takes resources to build anything. Would you try to build a house without any building materials? Would you start construction without any wood, nails, bricks, concrete or whatever else you were going to build your house out of? Of course not. Your housewarming party would just be a bunch of people standing in your yard eating egg salad while they talk about how you've lost your marbles. Just as when building a house, you need resources if you want to make a cute little human.

When a woman has horribly low resources, Mother Nature will often protect the would-be mother from troublesome issues by turning off the woman's ability to have a baby... and the menstrual cycle stops until her resources come back up. But we often punch Mother Nature in the face and work around her by using pharmaceutical hormones that keep the cycle regular. One of the most common underlying causes for a woman to experience irregular periods, or to go months at a time without a period, is a lack of proper digestion. That probably makes sense to you now that you've learned how digestion is what allows us to take the food we consume and turn it into life-sustaining resources. Once a woman can fully break down her food and pull the needed minerals out of what she's eating, her period commonly comes back.

We are taught that menopause is all about these crazy hormonal changes that take place in a woman's body when she reaches a certain point in her life, as if there is this clock in her body that's been waiting fifty years to go off; and once it does, craziness breaks loose. Hormones run amok, the menstrual cycle begins to go haywire, and "Why does my face feel like I'm on fire for forty seconds at a time?" Many women are advised to start cramming hormones into their bodies in order to "correct" this hormonal imbalance that comes with age. Why don't we ever stop to think that there might be a reason that these hormone levels are going crazy? Doesn't it make sense that, if the body is no longer receiving enough minerals and other nutrients it needs to function correctly, it might try to fix things on its own by raising hormone levels in a last-ditch effort to keep the body in a reproductive state? Once the body has tried every trick it has, the cycle will shut down and that individual will no longer have the ability to produce a child. This can be why many women enter menopause earlier than expected.

This also explains why pregnant women can have so many "loony" fits. We hear that this is due to all the crazy hormones flying around. I believe that could be true. However, couldn't these crazy hormonal changes be similar to those that come when the body is trying to figure out what to do about a lack of resources? In this regard, couldn't a lack of resources and hormonal changes be affecting those who are not pregnant as well? What if some people are creating mental issues by creating a nutrient deficiency with their extreme dieting techniques? Many may be creating these issues by just ignoring the task of taking care of the human body they live in. I have clients come to me all the time who will finally get around to eating a bag of corn chips around 2:30pm and won't eat again until dinner, or they skip dinner altogether. Do you really expect your body (much less your brain) to function on so little fuel?

If you have children and you send them to school without lunch money and no breakfast, and they are gone from 7am to 2 o'clock in the afternoon without eating, that could be 18 hours without food, depending on when they ate the night before. Child welfare will come and take your children away from you because that's flat out neglect. You wouldn't expect a child to excel with that type of neglect, so why would you expect a different outcome from your own body? In most cases, people who live this way don't really need therapy or a new direction in life; they need breakfast. Yes, digestion is important and that's always a priority, but how are you going to digest anything if you don't first insert it into your gullet?

So, Maybe I'm Not Fat Or Crazy, I'm Just Pregnant?

No. That's not what I said. But the circumstance of having a little human grow inside of you is an extreme that can show us how cravings increase as requirements escalate or as supply decreases. I'm hoping this illustrates how behavior can be affected by the nutrients you're supplying your body. It makes perfect sense to us when a pregnant woman says, "BRING ME CUCUMBERS WITH PEANUT BUTTER BEFORE I STOMP ON YOUR FACE!" We get it. Yet, her circumstances are just an exaggerated extreme of the same issues that can make you want to ball up on the floor and cry to old George Michael ballads.

If emotions seem to be elevated, use the same steps you took to get rid of cravings:

- Ensure digestion is working properly.
- Increase any supplements you are using to lift mineral content if you have an Electrolyte Deficiency Imbalance.
- Increase use of unrefined salt.
- Increase medium-carb foods.
- Consume appropriate fats and protein at every meal.

That Time Of The Month

While I'm on the topic of bodily situations that can arise for females, I want to mention the menstrual cycle. If cramps or horrible emotional roller coasters are part of your world every month, be sure to read my book, *Done With Menstrual Cramps*. For now, understand that your menstrual cycle requires an enormous amount of resources to complete the entire process. Therefore, when your period is approaching, expect resources to be low and the issues that can accompany low resources to be high. Take proper steps to ensure resources won't go too low during this time of the month.

Emotional Issues

The ability of your body chemistry to magnify many emotional issues does not mean that emotional issues do not exist—they do. Remember, improving chemistry doesn't fix all your problems, it can just make those problems easier for you to deal with. However, you still have to deal with them. I don't want to spend too much time on the subject because I don't want this to sound like a therapy session. I simply want you to know this... you can do it. Whatever it is, you can get past it. Why couldn't you? That doesn't mean it will be easy, it may not be easy at all. But the more difficult it is to get past, the bigger the reward will be on the other side.

I also want you to keep in mind that, no matter what you are dealing with, there is someone out there who would gladly trade problems with you. Appreciate where you are in your life because everything you're experiencing now is part of *your* journey and nobody can take that away from you. Be grateful for the life you're in and take responsibility for how it has turned out. That may be hard to do at first; but if you can take responsibility for your life, that can be enough to help you understand that you have the ability to change it.

"When you have exhausted all possibilities, remember this: You haven't."
                                                          - Thomas Edison

Get Support

Nobody said you need to get over emotional issues by yourself. What fun is that? Who are you going to high-five when you get there? Find support and don't be afraid to lean on that support. It's likely that they may need to help you as much as you need their help. If your emotional issues have to do with your weight, find a buddy who would like to lose weight too and take this journey together.   If everyone in your neighborhood is a skinny bitch, find people or communities online. On our site, www.DoneWithThatBooks.com, we have forums and communities for all types of issues; but when it comes to weight loss, I usually send people to the site for our documentary, www.WhyAmISoFatMovie.com. We have an amazing community there and you can find friends, ask questions and share your successes with others. It really can be a huge difference maker and it's totally free.

When Should I Weigh?

This is the best advice I can give people who deal with emotional issues connected to their weight. Most people will usually not listen to it and say I'll just do it my way, but the people who really follow this rule almost always do well.

Here's the advice: Don't weigh yourself... EVER!

"So, I don't count my calories and I don't weigh myself? Are you sure you're not just some moron that decided he wanted to write a book?" No, I'm not sure. But I do know weighing yourself constantly is one of the biggest mistakes I see new clients make.

You don't need to know what you weigh because you're not on a reality show where you win a million dollars for losing the most weight. The number on a scale is very misleading and it will really screw with your head. The thing that matters is how your clothes are fitting, especially your pants. Use that as your judge.

After all, how many times have you been in the middle of a weight loss program and gone without weighing yourself? And how many times have you succeeded to remove all the weight that you wanted to take off and keep it off? Exactly. Probably never on both accounts. Do something different. Just go by how you feel and how your clothes are fitting.

If you want to be more precise, measure your stomach right at your belly button first thing in the morning and mark that on the calendar. Then, measure your stomach again every two or three weeks. Don't do it more often than that because the body does not respond to what you did in the past day or two. That is not how weight loss works. Weight loss seems to work in cycles of seven to ten days. So, you could be doing everything perfectly for seven days, measure yourself and see no results and think that you need to change your approach. Had you just stuck with it for a few more days, the accumulative effect of that approach could have shown in another few days and you would have seen results. Don't mess with your head by measuring in the middle of your progress.

As far as actual weight goes, just weigh yourself when you start, mark it on the calendar, and you can weigh yourself every few months so you can tell your friends, "I lost thirty pounds, Dawg." Don't forget to take muscle into account for your weight. If you are working out and you are correcting any digestive issues and maybe you're adding more mineral to your intake, you now have the ability to build more muscle tissue. Muscle weighs more than fat, so you can actually go up on the scale, but still look and feel better. Your measurement around your stomach will never lie, but the scale will lie over and over again.

Again, some people don't take this advice seriously, but the ones who do, reach their goals more frequently and experience much less frustration along the way.

Low Potassium Issues

On top of emotional issues, if you start to feel a little loopy, clumsy or forgetful, this is great information to have. Potassium in the body is a mineral that allows the cells to communicate back to the brain. It's what closes the control loop. The brain says, "Okay, let's do this" and then everybody down in the body communicates back to the brain, "Okay, this is what happened." Without enough potassium, the "this is what happened" doesn't make it back to the brain. Beyond the lack of coordination with your muscle/brain communication, low potassium issues can also cause a lack of coordination in the endocrine system.

When there is a low-potassium issue, it's almost as if the body doesn't know what is going on since signals can't be properly transmitted. This can result in a variety of whacked-out testing numbers. pHs can be all over the board and your test results might not make much sense at all.

Low potassium issues can be easier to detect with equipment and techniques used by a professional health coach. However, here are some signs you can look for that commonly coincide with low potassium issues:

- Food seen in your stool
- Burping or bloating
- Significant digestive issues
- Clumsiness
- Absent-minded or forgetful

If these issues sound familiar, you may want to be skeptical of your testing results. That doesn't mean that you should supplement potassium. The next step I would take would be to work on any digestive issues. Once you improve digestion, and add protein to every meal, potassium can come into the system through your food. Good sources of extra potassium could be small green bananas, figs, a little blackstrap molasses, or orange juice. Just keep in mind that these are high-carb foods, and high-carb foods are not always the best idea when trying to lose weight.

Be Patient

Results make it easy to be optimistic and keep emotions positive. However, it's important to understand that, when taking steps to move chemistry, most results will not show up immediately. That's not how the body works. You can't take a supplement or eat a specific food and expect your chemistry to be different an hour later, or even the next day. In that same line of thinking, you can't see a major change in your numbers and look at what you just did and think that was responsible. You can't say to yourself, "Well, I just watched an old episode of *Bewitched* and now my blood pressure is better." That's not how it works. You want the changes to your body to move slowly, just like agriculture does. Let me tell you a story to illustrate what I mean.

I was living in Florida and touring professionally as a comic. I was on a three-month trip all over the West Coast and still had a girlfriend on the East Coast. While I was working a week in Vegas, she flew out to see me. We were sitting at the buffet when we heard over the intercom, "Phone call for Mr. Knievel, Mr. Evel Knievel." We laughed at how someone must have gotten a hold of the intercom and was playing a joke. But that night, Evel Knievel came to my show and sat in the back of the room with my girlfriend. This part has nothing to do with my illustration, I just like to talk about Evel Knievel. The point of the story is that my girlfriend and I broke up on that trip. Not because she wanted me to be dreamier like Evel Knievel, but because with the long time away, we had just grown apart. The split was amicable but as I dropped her off at the airport, she couldn't stop crying. I was sad that we were splitting up, but I just wasn't emotional about it.

I returned to the airport the next morning for my flight back home, as my West Coast tour had ended and I missed all my rednecks in Florida. I got on the plane and sat in the middle seat between two very large men. Normally, when you sit down on a plane, you might share a few pleasantries or at least say, "Hi." For one reason or another, none of us said a word. I may have been silent just because both guys were a lot taller than me and I could tell I was going to lose the armrest battle. About an hour into the flight, the cart started moving down the aisle to serve breakfast.

The stewardess, or sky frolicker, or whatever the current politically correct name is, set my breakfast on my fold-out tray. I looked down to see two pieces of french toast, cut in half, with a sliced-up pear in the middle. Pears were my girlfriend's favorite food. I looked down at the plate for about 30 seconds before tears started running down my face. By the time the air waitress had moved the cart down the aisle, I was sobbing like an eight-year-old girl who just accidentally smashed the cassette for her *Annie* soundtrack. It was full-on uncontrollable sobbing. Not cool. It lasted for more than a few minutes before the guy sitting to my right finally looked over and asked, "Are you okay?" I paused for a moment, collected myself, looked straight ahead and said to him with a trembling voice, "I just really like french toast." The guy to my left looked over to the guy to my right for a brief second, they both looked straight ahead just long enough to let what I said soak in, then we all went back to eating our breakfast and nobody said another word for the rest of the flight.

Do you see my point? I'm thinking that maybe you don't, but it's still a good story. My sobbing was not a result of the pears I just saw. There were layers upon layers of events, emotions and circumstances that led to my making a complete idiot out of myself on the plane that morning. That's how your body works. Just because you're trying to improve one imbalance doesn't mean that many layers of imbalances, emotions and chemistry are not being affected in many ways. With that in mind, try not to view a piece of information merely as cause and effect. It is often much more intricate than that and results will often take longer than you want them to take. Be patient. Your health is not an episode of *Miami Vice*. Everything will not be resolved in forty-five minutes.

Calling In A Professional

I've already gone on and on about how tricky this process can be. Always remember that you are educating yourself about your body. The human body is just about the most amazing mechanism out there. (Other than a slinky. I just don't see how it does that thing down the stairs.) While you're working to better understand your body, keep in mind that *nobody* totally understands the human body. It's way too complicated. Remember that understanding these imbalances is complex enough, but when you start to realize that one imbalance on top of another can begin to change how the whole system is running, it can be a lot to sort through. I know there are people who will totally change their life, or lose an incredible amount of weight, by simply improving their digestion or a slight imbalance here or there, but a percentage of you will really need help from a professional to see major progress. Remember, you still need to be able to deal with any emotional issues that could slow this journey so sometimes having a professional guide you through the scientific parts can be a load off of you. The best part about plugging yourself into *The Coalition* and using their tracking tools is that you will be laying the groundwork in case you need to bring in a health coach to help you. When you contact *The Coalition* to find a professional in your area, and you begin to work with that person, *The Coalition* can then attach your account to that health coach. The coach will then be able to see all of your progress charts and how your chemistry has been moving with the efforts you have been putting in.

Presenting a new health coach with data that you have already been tracking can be a tremendous jump-start—not to mention the fact that you will understand your body enough now to have an intelligent conversation with the person who is guiding you in your education about your body. Unlike a doctor visit where you might not have a clue what he's talking about or why he's suggesting the things he is suggesting, if you've read this book and you've been monitoring your chemistry on *The Coalition*, you will be miles ahead of the game. It will be so much easier for you to be a participant in your own health.

Wha'd He Say?

In this chapter, you learned:

- A lack of nutrients can create emotional roller coaster issues.
- Many people don't need therapy, they need breakfast.
- Don't weigh yourself too frequently. Use measurements or how your clothes are fitting to monitor your progress.
- If you're feeling loopy, clumsy or forgetful, you may be dealing with low potassium issues.
- Be patient.
- If you need help from a professional health coach, get it. You don't need to do this alone.

CHAPTER TWELVE

What Else Can Help?

Improving digestion, curbing your cravings and making adjustments to reduce insulin spikes from sugar and carb consumption are your biggest initial steps. Those are the three things that are going to bring the most number of people the greatest results. That doesn't mean that some other step in this book isn't going to be your most effective change, it just means that for most people, those initial three things are key. Correcting imbalances is the next major step. Now let's look at what else can bring you closer to your weight loss goals.

Starvation Mode - Don't Skip Breakfast

"You can find the time to eat breakfast, or you can find the time to buy bigger pants."
                                                                    - Me

By skipping breakfast, you go too many waking hours without food and your body can actually go into starvation mode. Your body doesn't know that you're just too busy to eat. It thinks that you're going into a time of drought and you may not eat for days. So, it will slow down your bodily functions and your metabolism and begin to store whatever it can as fat so that it will have a future fuel source if needed. If you do this a few days in a row, once you finally do eat, your body says, "Oh, here's some stuff I can store for more fuel later since times have been so lean lately." You really need to eat at least three meals a day if you want to lose weight. Three meals with two snacks is the best way to go so that you have smaller meals more frequently. If you're waking up late and still eating within an hour or so of waking, that can be considered your breakfast. Even a protein shake for breakfast would at least be some form of nutrition. But out of all your daily meals, breakfast is the most important.

If you're normally nauseous in the morning and have no appetite, I'm not going to require you to cram something in your face. You may be able to make adjustments to improve that nausea and then breakfast won't be such a bad idea. If you're already working on digestion and you're using Beet Flow to improve your bile flow (as described in chapter three), this will often improve nausea issues. Coffee suppositories or coffee enemas can also be useful tools when trying to move bile that may be difficult to get moving.

Water

Water is a pretty big deal when discussing the toxicity level in a human body. After all, water is one of the biggest components that allows the human body to wash toxins out. Keep in mind that a toxic person is often an overweight person. The body is 70% water and is based on aqueous chemistry; it doesn't work too well without the aqueous. If you're not drinking enough water, you're trying to wash your windows with mud. I'm about to completely yell at you for the lack of water that you drink. But before I do, know that I am yelling at only about half of you.

If an Electrolyte Deficiency Imbalance showed up on your *Imbalance Guide*, you might not qualify to drink more water. Water not only washes out junk, it can wash out minerals as well. If you have very few minerals in the system, increasing your water intake may just wash out the small amount of good stuff that you do have. If you're a person who has low blood pressure, and you avoid drinking a lot of water because it makes you feel lousy, now you know why. You just lowered your blood pressure more.

That does not mean that you don't need that water. You absolutely do. If you continue to avoid water, problems are headed your way. You do, however, need to bring up your mineral content by improving digestion, adding unrefined salt and using any supplements that could lift blood pressure. As you do this, you can begin to increase your water little by little. Be mindful, though, that if you start to feel lousy, check your blood pressure to see if it has gone down because you may be increasing water intake faster than you are lifting your mineral content.

For those of you with an Electrolyte Excess Imbalance, water can be your best friend. If your blood pressure is high, odds are great that you're not drinking enough pure water. Still, all water is not created equal. Since the body uses water to help remove junk, don't you think it would be a good idea to drink water that is not filled with junk in the first place? If your car is covered in dirt, does it make sense to wash it off with water filled with smashed up chocolate chip cookies? Your car wouldn't get cleaner; you would just be replacing one layer of junk with another layer of junk. With this mind, don't view all liquid drinks as water. If you're stirring flavored powder containing sugar or artificial sweeteners into your water, or making coffee with your water, that doesn't count as water. Water is water.

Note: If more water makes your stool too loose, you may have a Catabolic Imbalance so check your numbers to see if they lean toward a Catabolic Imbalance.

Avoid Soda

Soda has different meanings or connotations in different areas of the country. I'm talking about carbonated, flavored drinks—soda pop. I advocate seltzer water or sparkling water to many clients with slower breath rates (say, below 10 breaths per minute) and especially if they're having panic attacks. Breathing into a paper bag increases CO_2 in the system and allows oxygen to be released to the brain. This can ease some panic attacks. Seltzer water accomplishes the same thing without the obvious inappropriateness of breathing into a paper bag. If someone is having a panic attack, Pepsi-Cola has more acid than Coca-Cola and I advocate Pepsi for the panic attack if seltzer or sparkling water is not available at the quick stop gas station.

Beyond this handy use, the average soft drinks are just a transport system for artificial sweeteners and chemicals that your body can't process. The worst part is that they also contain phosphates that have been proven to block your body's ability to assimilate nutrients. So, basically, any food that you eat along with a diet soda is not being assimilated optimally by your body. Incredible, isn't it? That affects most of the country. This info gives you some clues why so many in this country are overweight with diabetes, heart disease or cancer. Our bodies aren't getting the nutrients they need to function properly.

Quitting soda can be very hard for some people. You can actually get withdrawal symptoms because the chemicals act like a drug. But once you get past eight or nine days without any soda at all, you should find it much easier to quit drinking soda completely. Your body will start to forget that it can use those chemicals and sweeteners to thicken your blood—and your cravings can stop altogether.

Most people think that they're making the healthy choice by drinking diet. In my opinion, the only ingest-able substance that you can put in your body that is worse for you than diet soda is a jelly doughnut, and that's only because it's fried. The artificial sweeteners used in diet soda are directly linked to so many brain and mental issues that it's hard to keep up. Once my clients get past the initial difficult week of giving up soda, most of them lose at least five pounds; and nearly half of their nagging symptoms simply go away.

My clients with a low mineral content in their bodies seem to love soda the most and, just like smoking, have the hardest time giving it up. Soda has syrup in it that makes it thicker so the taste sticks on the tongue longer. This syrup also makes your blood thicker and raises your blood pressure. This is one of the reasons people crave it so much and have a hard time quitting. The body can use it to thicken your blood and buffer low salts and low sugars.

I have even read that, when many companies ship the concentrated syrup that goes into soda to give it that flavor and texture people can't seem to live without, the companies actually have to post a "Transporting Hazardous Substance" sign on their trucks. And we just dilute this stuff with some carbonated water and drink it? Amazing.

Removing soda from your diet can better help you digest your food, use the nutrients in that food, and can help every aspect of your body. For many people, nothing in this book will improve their health more than losing the soda. When you're drinking soda, not only are you bringing in junk, you're also *not* drinking water... the thing your body really needs.

Lose The Artificial Sweeteners

Anytime you see "Sugar Free" on a package, you can almost guarantee it has some type of artificial sweetener in it. That's how it still tastes good even though they took all the sugar out. The problem is that these artificial sweeteners are just that: ARTIFICIAL. Some artificial sweeteners market themselves as a natural sweetener and say that they are "made from sugar." That is fiction. They are just as bad for you as aspartame. Because it's artificial, the body can't recognize it and process it properly. Now, it just becomes a toxin that the body has to deal with.

There are also a lot of products out now sweetened with agave and honey and such. These are still high in sugars and carbs, but they are natural and better than using an artificial sweetener or refined sugar. I don't view these products as toxic; but since they can spike insulin levels, just like sugar can, I try to avoid them. Inositol, inulin, xylitol, and lo han guo are not horrible and these products will not spike insulin levels. Xylitol comes from either corn or birch trees. I'm not much of a fan of anything that comes from corn, so I prefer to use the variety that comes from birch trees, if I use it at all. I'm not a fan of sucralose.

The only sweetener that I honestly view as healthy is stevia. It's just an herb and doesn't have any effect on insulin levels. Stevia is pro-anabolic, so I don't recommend any severe anabolics using large amounts of stevia. But once you improve an Anabolic Imbalance, introducing small amounts of stevia would likely be okay.

I will be honest, however, and tell you that nobody in his right mind could possibly just start using stevia. Disgusting. But here's the trick and, trust me, I have not had one single person who actually followed through with this who didn't say, "Holy cow, you're right, I really like it!" The weird thing is that they all said, "Holy Cow." Weird, huh? Anyway, you can't just start using stevia when your body is accustomed to sugar and artificial sweeteners. The trick is to use whatever you use now, and add just a little bit of stevia. You won't even taste it at first. Then, the next time, you add a little more stevia until you have it at about half and half. Then, you just start using less of your sweetener until it's gone. By that time, your taste buds will have changed and you will have acquired a taste for stevia. After you get used to it, you will like it. My advice is to get the flavored drops they sell at most health food stores so you get a little bonus flavor.

I do not have any financial interest in "Nu Naturals" Stevia, but I understand the stevia leaf has two molecules in it that give us the sensation of sweet. One of those molecules has a bitter aftertaste. This particular brand is made only from the one molecule that does not have that bitterness.

Use Unrefined Salt (Sea Salt)

For people who have low mineral content and low blood pressure, a quality sea salt can literally change their life. Sea salt is, in essence, minerals from the sea. It also contains a chloride ion that is necessary for your body to make its own HCL. Without this chloride ion, people can't make enough HCL to properly digest their food.

Some people tell me that they don't like salt. Usually this is because they have associated decreased health with using salt so they begin to avoid it. However, as your body realizes, "Hey, we can really use this stuff for a lot of functions," your taste buds will change, you will begin to really like the taste and you'll even crave it.

"Flower of the Ocean" by Celtic Sea Salt is my favorite brand, but don't feel like this is your only option. Any unrefined salt or unrefined sea salt should bring you some benefits. Redmond Real Salt is a popular unrefined salt used by many health coaches. Some feel that, since the sea is polluted, it is better to use a mined salt like Redmond Real Salt. Even if you're out at a restaurant and don't have any unrefined salt available to you, normal table salt could help you out of a rough spot if you're experiencing a lot of sugar cravings.

If you can't find Celtic Sea Salt or Redmond Real Salt, most Himalayan sea salts are also good in a pinch, in my opinion. If you think I was making an idiotic pun-like joke with the "pinch" in reference to salt, I will be furious.

Fiber

If you make the change to eating more real food, rather than processed junk, odds are great that you will already be increasing your fiber. This is very important when it comes to weight loss. Fiber helps the body gather up the garbage and push it out the back door.

As crucial as fiber can be for your health, that doesn't mean that all high-fiber foods are good choices. In chapter five I taught you how to find the fiber content on a nutrition label allowing you to calculate the active carbs. Be sure to do this when you're looking for foods higher in fiber. Most foods that are advertised as "high fiber" also have a ridiculous amount of carbs in them. You do want more fiber, but you don't want it to come with spiking your insulin levels—so always remember to look at the active carbs.

All green leafy vegetables are excellent sources of good fiber. I also like my clients to use fiber supplements. It's so easy to pop a few fiber capsules when you wake up and before you go to bed; you add a big fiber boost with very little effort.

Knowledge

Knowledge is power, and can help more than just about anything when it comes to weight loss and your health. However, as important as it is to gain knowledge, it is also important to avoid knowledge that may not be so accurate. Clinical trials can be a very misleading source of information.

A new clinical trial reported recently that high blood pressure rates would drop 68% if they would put *Alf* back on the air. I'm pretty sure I'm the only person who has ever written that statement, but it makes my point that we will believe just about anything that was discovered by a clinical trial. It's my opinion that these clinical trials are often the origin of bad information. Once you understand how every individual is different, and no two people have the same chemistry, or are able to process foods, emotions or pollutants the exact same way, we begin to see that giving a room full of people the same supplement, drug, or forcing them all to wear a Fonzie jacket, really doesn't prove anything.

When we look at results from a clinical trial, the only consistency we know across the board is that all participants were human. These days, it can even be hard to tell gender. We really don't know any of the important factors about these clinical trial participants. We don't know if they are digesting their food correctly. We don't know if they even have the ability to assimilate whatever substance they are testing. It's all a shot in the dark. When the numbers turn out that 59% of headache sufferers improved when they ate a peanut butter and jelly sandwich at 5:30 PM every day, suddenly the world comes to a halt at 5:30 to spread a little Jif on some bread. What about the other 41% of the participants? Even if they experienced an increase in symptom severity, the trial still says PBJs help the majority of headache sufferers. Unless we're looking at a person's individual chemistry, and then taking stock of how a substance can move that chemistry while it creates changes to those symptoms, we're just cramming a hundred people in a dark closet, throwing in a Freddy Krueger mask, and then counting the number of people who pee their pants. How is this science?

The only thing we do know about a clinical trial is that it was bought and paid for by somebody. Some company (most often a pharmaceutical manufacturer) put up the money to fund this trial (and trials are not cheap) because they were hoping to create a specific result that would help them sell a drug, procedure or substance.

The lesson here about clinical trials is this: Even a Fonzie jacket can't make everybody look cool, and don't make decisions about your health based on the results of a group of people whose chemistry was unknown before the trial and remains unknown after the trial. Without a clear, chemistry-driven baseline to start from, how can you come to any conclusions about whatever it was they were testing?

Simma Down Now

People always say stress is bad for you but they never say why. Anger, stress, frustration and all those emotions seen as danger (thereby justifying a need for energy) can cause the body to lift sugar levels and hormones in your body. All these chemicals are just more garbage your body has to deal with. It's like eating a Ding Dong. When you eat processed junk food, your body has to deal with those chemicals and sugars. The chemicals created from your stress have to be dealt with by the body too. Your body can do only so much at once. If it is dealing with chemicals from stress at a time that it could have been removing some toxin that was brought in from a food or pollutant, now these other toxins can end up being stored as fat since the body is busy elsewhere. Remember how the body takes junk that it can't deal with and shoves it into fat cells? This makes the toxins inert and "harmless" to the body. In this regard, can stress make you fat? In a roundabout way, I guess it can.

Many scientific papers have been written about the effects cortisol can have on body fat. It appears that stress can increase levels of the hormone, cortisol, which signals the body to store more fat. Whether cortisol is really the culprit or not is unimportant, in my opinion. When you believe that something like cortisol is the problem, you may try to buy supplements that reduce your cortisol levels and then you continue the same horrible behavior that got you here. I'd rather see you take steps to reduce your stress and work on the root of the problem instead of always trying to cheat your way to easier results. I know. I've done this myself. Throughout three years of high school Spanish class, my friends and I all cheated off of this kid who spoke fluent Spanish. I got all A's and B's, but on my trip to Mexico, I couldn't speak a lick of Spanish.

Under stress, your body will also take blood and energy away from the digestive processes to deal with the immediate threat (the threat being whatever is causing you stress). Your body doesn't know that you're stressed merely because you're stuck in traffic. To your body, your interpretation of stress is equal to, "We're being chased by a lion so create chemicals that will help us get away from a lion." Under stress, your body will also push more glucose into the bloodstream to be used as immediate energy. When glucose levels get high, insulin has to increase to handle that glucose and we already know that can lead to more stored fat. Look at that, stress is making you fat again. For crying out loud, calm down!

I don't know how stressed you actually are. If it's a lot, start thinking about ways that you can process these stressful situations in your life in a more calming manner. Or see if you can find a little time for yourself to relax in some way, even if it's just stopping and taking a deep breath a few times a day. The body is already under a lot of stress. Not only is it stressed to remove toxins and pollutants, or fight off invaders that have set up a college party town in your body, stress can also be induced by a lack of resources. I've talked a lot in this book about different circumstances that can result in a lack of resources within the body. Well, a lack of resources is a stress to the body. "How am I going to pay $800 worth of bills with $15?" That's the type of situation your body has to figure out when it needs a large number of resources and there aren't enough coming in due to a lack of digestion or poor diet choices.

Diet choices! There's another possible stress to the body. Do you really think your body was made to consume squirt cheese? This is not food. This is not what your body was made to run on. The things we call food these days are enough to stress out any human body. Let's say you worked on an assembly line and your job was to pick up the square pegs off the conveyor belt and place them in the boxes. One day, instead of square pegs on the conveyor belt, you started seeing balloon animals. Your supervisor is nowhere to be seen. You know that if you get behind again you're going to be fired, so you just have to do the best you can at cramming the inflated poodle balloons into boxes that were made for square pegs. This would be stressful. This is what many of our bodies go through every day. The body has to figure out this scramble of, "How do I take this substance that does not contain any redeeming nutritional value and process it with a digestive system that was made to process real food?" Help your body and eat something that comes from the earth instead of from a package in a vending machine.

Wha'd He Say?

In this chapter, you learned:

- Eat breakfast.
- If you have an Electrolyte Deficiency Imbalance, you may need more water, but you first need to qualify to drink more water by increasing your mineral content.
- If you have an Electrolyte Excess Imbalance, you need to drink more water. No, really... drink more water.
- Soda is not water and soda is not good.
- Artificial sweeteners can create weight gain just as much as, if not more than, sugar.
- Unrefined salt can change your life, especially if you have an Electrolyte Deficiency Imbalance.
- Fiber is an easy way to cheat and push more junk out of your body.
- Clinical trials can often be misleading due to the fact that we don't know the digestive capacity or the body chemistry of those participating in the trial.
- CALM DOWN!!!

CHAPTER THIRTEEN

Conflicting Advice Everywhere:
What The Heck Should I Eat?

I know!!! It couldn't possibly be more confusing out in the world of weight loss, right? If you try to listen to a nutritionist, follow the most popular diet book on the market and read a fitness magazine at the same time, you're likely going to be pulled in three different directions. I'm hoping you're starting to realize why this occurs. I'm hoping you understand that there is no diet that is right for every person and this is why nobody can agree on anything.

In chapter fourteen I list foods that can be beneficial for improving specific imbalances and, in chapter fifteen, I provide you with sample meal plans. You'll then be able to incorporate the foods that may be optimal for how your body is operating into a meal plan designed for weight loss.

In this chapter I give you general guidelines, tell you about foods that anyone hoping to lose weight should avoid, and answer the most common questions that people ask me about food. And no, I don't want fries with that.

What About Meat?

I think I get this question more often than just about any other. Is meat healthy? So here's the breakdown:

Chemicals, Hormones And Antibiotics

If you're buying meat at your local grocery store or if you're eating at the average restaurant or if you're eating at just about any fast food place, you're likely paying for junk meat that was mass-produced. When farmers mass-produce in this manner, they often keep the animals in small cages and feed them the cheapest type of food they can come up with so they can make a profit. Keep in mind this farmer has a competitor down the street trying to sell meat to the same large corporation cheaper, and the bean counters on Wall Street are going to tell the corporation to buy the cheaper product with no idea how it became cheaper or where the quality went. Often times, these animals are eating foods that their stomachs were not even designed to eat. The result from this upbringing is frequent illness and a lot of dying animals—animals that could have been sold to make a profit. So what does Mr. Farmer do? He pumps the animals full of antibiotics, drugs, hormones and other chemicals to keep them alive long enough to reach a size that will make them profitable.

If you pump cows or chickens full of drugs and antibiotics, they don't just poop that out at the end of the day. Those drugs go into their tissues and guess where those tissues end up… yes, right in your cheeseburger. That's why the antibiotic wonder drugs of 30 years ago are beginning to work less and less. We all take in such a small dose of antibiotics on a daily basis through the animal protein we eat that the bad bugs (little creatures that invade our bodies and cause havoc) build up a tolerance to these drugs until the drugs are no longer effective. So, is meat bad? If this is the meat you're eating, yes it is.

Digesting Meat

Another problem with meat is that well over half of the population doesn't have their digestion working correctly. I have seen clients correct their amazingly horrific symptoms and conditions by just correcting their digestion, more than any other issue. Like I talked about in chapter three, one of our digestive processes is the acid that is formed in our stomach to help break down protein. But if you're not making enough acid, that meat doesn't even start to get broken down. To understand how this is bad, try the following trick: Take a big bag of carrots and put them in a garbage can outside your house. Take another garbage can and fill it with raw meat. Let them sit there for about a week and go back, take the lid off and stick your head in each garbage can. Let me know which one smells worse. Which one did a better job of rotting, fermenting, attracting bugs and other crazy chemical reactions? If you don't want to do this experiment, I'll let you know: It's the meat.

So, just like in the trash can, if meat doesn't get properly digested, it will rot, ferment and create nasty chemicals that can throw off your body's balance and create issues, conditions and "disease." But that doesn't mean that the real problem is the meat itself, it's just the fact that you can't break it down. Without digestion, that meat becomes something else—something else that you don't want in your body.

When Is Meat Healthy?

Does this help explain why so many authorities say that meat is bad for you? Why some vegetarians feel so much better when they stop eating meat? If their digestion isn't working well, they will feel much better "not digesting" vegetables than they did "not digesting" meat. Plus, if they were eating standard store- or restaurant-bought meat, they would feel better when they stopped putting all those drugs and chemicals into their systems. Nonetheless, this doesn't prove that meat is really bad for you. If you are a person who actually has your digestion working properly and you buy meat or eggs that come from organic, free-range animals, animal protein can be a very healthy, and even necessary, part of your diet. With all the "studies" they do on eating meat and diseases that come from doing so, have you ever heard of a study using organic, free-range meats? It never happens. Have you ever heard of a study using only people with their digestion working properly? Of course not. 90% of the people with bad digestion don't even know that they have bad digestion.

The truth is, a lot of people really need animal protein. Here's how it works: Everything on the planet that eats, for the most part, is doing so to bring in nutrients and minerals so their body can function correctly. Well, these nutrients and minerals actually come from the Earth's soil. But as humans, we can't just pick up dirt and eat it because our bodies don't have the ability to process those nutrients. However, if we eat the plants that eat those minerals and nutrients from the soil (so to speak), we have an easier time translating those nutrients to something we can use in our bodies. If we take that a step further and eat the meat from the animals that ate those plants, the nutrients and minerals are even closer to a state that we can use.

Does this mean that you have to eat meat? Not necessarily. You can get a lot of the important nutrients you would get from meat by using the correct supplements. What it does mean is this: You don't have to stop eating meat to be healthy; and if you don't eat meat, you do need to supplement nutrients so you are getting the important nutrients that you're missing. But as long as your digestion is working correctly, the only thing left to do is buy good, quality meats and eggs that are organic, free-range and hormone-free. To the person with good digestion, everything is food; to the person with poor digestion, nothing is food. To quote my own book, "Diet is what a person eats but nutrition is what the cells see."

Vegan / Vegetarian

This is a fun section because I know people become defensive when they see the heading. "Is he going to make me just eat weeds?" or "Is he going to speak poorly of me and my vegan cohorts?" No matter what side of the fence some people may stand on, most simply don't want to hear about the other side. But you've figured out by now that I'm really not that nice and I'm probably going to end up bashing both sides, tear down the fence, and build a bonfire where we'll roast a pig and drink wheatgrass juice, all at the same party.

First of all, I will say that I was vegan for nearly two years; and it really is not as difficult as you may think. It's just a matter of creating new habits and learning new recipes. Everything else is just life and putting food choices into that life. (I don't know if that sentence makes any sense but I kinda like it for some reason.) If you have chosen to be a vegan or vegetarian because of your love for animals, or you hate the idea of eating anything with a face, or your religion tells you to "praise all creatures who can poop," or anything like that, then I suggest continuing that path. If that is what makes you happy, I won't argue with you. I, on the other hand, became a vegan because I thought that was the healthiest choice to make. Turns out... not so true.

When you first start eating vegetarian, you will often feel better, have better energy and you may lose weight as well. Let's look at why that happens. First of all, if you're eating the wrong kinds of meat or your digestion is not working well enough to break down the meat you were eating (as discussed under *What About Meat?* earlier in this chapter), then by eliminating that meat, you are taking away a burden that your body was dealing with while you were consuming meat. Now that your body doesn't have to deal with the chemicals, hormones and drugs that were in the meat, or your body doesn't have to try to digest a food that it doesn't have the resources to break down properly, now it can turn its attention to removing junk from the body. Anytime digestion is not working properly, vegetables will break down much easier than meat. By making the switch to a vegetarian diet, you also free up more resources, resulting in more energy. Vegetables also contain nutrients that will help bind to acids and other toxins, allowing them to be safely removed from the body, resulting in weight loss. Since you are now eating less meat, you will obviously be eating more vegetables so you will receive more of the benefits from these types of nutrients. Pretty good deal, huh? Well, that's not really the whole story.

Now pay attention because I'm about to sound smart. In the same way that vegetables contain nutrients that you need (nutrients you can't get from any other sources), so does animal protein. When you first stop eating meat, your body has a reserve of these nutrients that can be utilized for a period of time until you run out. Therefore, in the beginning, you're not overworking your digestive system by trying to eat meat that you can't digest, you're getting more good vegetable nutrients that your body needs in order to remove waste and toxins, and you still have a reserve of animal-based nutrients that your body can pull from as needed. It's all good, you feel great and you wonder why you didn't become a vegetarian a long time ago. As time passes, however, you begin to run out of the reserves of animal-based nutrients and you run into trouble. Your body will even begin to break down your own tissues to pull the nutrients required, as if you are the animal that your body is eating. As people begin to feel worse, they don't even consider the fact that they need animal protein because they felt so great in the beginning when they stopped eating it. Do you see how the confusion sets in?

Is eating vegetarian healthy for a lot of people? Sure. Especially if their digestion isn't working well enough to break down meat and the meat is just going to rot and ferment in their stomachs. But the truly optimal thing to do is to fix your digestion so you can actually break down the meat you eat, then, eat meat that is free of hormones, drugs and disease. Eating a diet that is far heavier in vegetables than meat is always the best plan. But I find that most people, at least in the long run, do need some form of meat (even if it's just eggs) in order to be fully healthy. If you are some type of ovo-vegetarian, or fresh water fish that begin with "t" vegetarian, or some new-fangled name that makes you feel more important than the rest of us, that may be a good route for you. Including some type of animal protein like fish, eggs, or chicken (even dairy can work well for many people), can be enough for a lot of people to get by on a vegetarian diet. If it isn't, you can always use supplements to try to fill in the missing pieces. That being said, just taking B12 is not enough to fill in the gaps. Animal proteins contain amino acids and nutrient cofactors that cannot be replaced with a B12 capsule.

Vegetarianism And Weight Gain

Here's the real problem many vegetarians face: When you're eating less meat, you're eating less protein; and the protein you are eating is most commonly some type of processed vegetarian protein. So, if you are eating an ample amount of protein, it's probably a processed non-food that you are consuming. Also, when you eat less protein, that means you are likely eating more carbohydrates. More carbohydrates means that you are going to spike your insulin levels which can lead to weight gain. Yes, as a new vegetarian, you can begin to lose weight after the initial release of toxins that were building up from undigested meat and chemicals you were consuming from eating the wrong meat. However, a lot of vegetarians have a hard time losing weight in the long run because they are eating so many complex carbohydrates that they block their body's ability to burn any stored fat as fuel.

Balance is always the best route.
Correcting digestion is always the first step.
It will always be that way.

Organic vs. Conventional

I'm going to share a couple viewpoints on this topic and one of them may surprise you. As a way to recognize natural products as being the best in their field, my company, www.ShapeYou.com, developed a program called the GearAwards. Manufacturers send us their products in hopes of winning one of our awards. With this program, I get to see a lot of new merchandise before it hits the market and I will say this: Nothing is more popular right now than slapping the word "organic" on a label. This is where the market is going. More people than ever are realizing the importance of buying organic. Since I like to hang out with the cool kids, let me first explain why buying organic is a good thing before I share the other viewpoint.

Wikipedia (which is always correct, right?) lists the definition of Organic Food as "foods that are produced using methods that do not involve modern synthetic inputs such as synthetic pesticides and chemical fertilizers, do not contain genetically modified organisms, and are not processed using irradiation, industrial solvents, or chemical food additives." If you combine this definition with what I wrote about chemicals and hormones found in meats, you can probably guess what I'm going to say next. When we eat foods that are filled with all these chemicals, where do you think those chemicals go? They go right into us, into our machines that we count on to carry us around all day. Just like any other synthetic or toxic substance that I've covered in this book, when these materials enter the body, the alarm sounds and the question is asked, "What the heck is this stuff?" When the human body encounters something that it doesn't recognize, it wants to send it out of the system. In essence, it becomes a problem to be dealt with.

People are starting to get the idea that if you're going to make the effort to eat healthier and swap out your corn chips for broccoli, it might be a good idea to make sure the broccoli isn't loaded with harmful chemicals. Otherwise, you might as well stick with the corn chips.

Since the market is asking for organic products, organic products are starting to show up in places you might not expect to see them. It's fantastic that America's eyes are being opened to how harmful our despicable, almost bionic, farming methods have become. But it does freak me out a little to think about how some of the bigger corporations may take this organic foundation and start to figure out how to cut corners and save a buck. Until then, I will continue to enjoy the increased variety of organic foods available.

Fresh vs. Frozen

One thing that may surprise you is that frozen organic vegetables can sometimes be even better for you than the fresh produce. Most of the fresh produce you find in a store was picked days or even weeks ago and has been making its way through the handling process to show up on the shelf where you can buy it. During this time, the vegetable can cannibalize itself to stay alive. If you look at the bottom of a broccoli stem, you can often see where it has started to become hollow from the broccoli eating itself. Also, fresh produce is often picked before it is ripened so it can ripen during its travels. If the produce is picked early, its ability to absorb minerals was stunted by an early dismissal from the fields. Now this vegetable is not as dense with nutrients as it could have been if it matured properly.

Frozen vegetables are ripened on the vine and picked and frozen right away so all of that mineral stays intact. Plus, now you have the convenience of keeping vegetables in your freezer that are good for you.

Of course, the best way to go is to grow your own food or buy it at a trusted farmer's market where the produce was picked fresh. Not everyone has these options; but if you do, it's worth the extra effort or cost involved.

Organic Does Not Mean Healthy

I see this a lot. People will adapt to some new form of eating, whether it be vegan, organic, gluten-free, etc., and they think that as long as a food is gluten-free or organic, it must be healthy. Guess what? That's not even close to being true. If you make an organic candy bar, it's still a candy bar. Using organic ingredients doesn't change the fact that it's a pile of sugar that is going to spike your insulin levels. I will say that I do applaud the effort of some companies to remove chemicals, preservatives, artificial sweeteners and such, and make a sweet snack for kids that is sweetened by more natural things, like agave, honey or raw sugar. I applaud it, but that doesn't mean I would eat it or tell my clients to eat it. It is simply a step in the right direction. I appreciate the companies that are trying to provide an alternative to the submarine shaped non-food snack cakes that I grew up on. I have even been known to give a company an award for their attempts, even if it's a product I wouldn't eat myself. It's still something that is at least a 50% improvement over what else is out there, and I commend them on their efforts.

Organic just means that it doesn't include harmful chemicals. It's not a magic wand that automatically makes any food good for you. You still need to make good choices. Yes, by eating organic you can eliminate some detrimental materials from entering your body, just do so intelligently. (I just had to use the spell corrector on the word "intelligently." Is that only funny to me?)

Organic Does Not Mean Nutritious

Here is the viewpoint that is often missed: Our food is horrible. I mean, it contains a fraction of the nutrients that it did sixty years ago. Our "franken-farming" methods are making it possible for us to create beautiful looking produce that contains almost no minerals whatsoever. This is generally done by using chemicals that allow the plant to grow without the intended mineral. This concern is not restricted to conventional farming methods by any means. Organic farming restrictions don't impose any rules on whether or not the soil needs to be properly replenished, or even if the soil contained appropriate amounts of mineral in the first place. This is where the mineral in our food comes from—the plant pulls it out of the soil. If the soil has been depleted, and if proper methods have not been utilized to allow the earth to replenish itself, those organic crops are going to be missing nutrients.

You probably know that there is a variety of pests that can destroy farmers' crops. It is said that the mineral that exists within a plant is what helps the plant fight off pests that can destroy it. That is why conventional farming methods require pesticides—the lack of mineral in those crops has rendered them helpless against invaders. This is the basis of my optimism about organic farming. I like to believe that an organic crop must at least have enough mineral in it to survive without pesticides. I do not know that this is a fact, this is just an optimistic view that I hold on organic farming. However, my optimism does not mean that organic farmers are properly replenishing the soil. I agree that, when buying organic, we at least know that we are eliminating some poisons. It just doesn't mean that we're getting everything that is intended to be in that food. That organic food could still be lacking the nutrition that we are seeking. Studies have indicated that organic produce does contain more mineral than conventionally grown, but there is no way to show that this is true and consistent with all organic produce. The level of mineral within a food is more dependent on the soil it came from, rather than the organic label on the product itself.

You Mean I Can Eat That?

The following two chapters will dig further into specific foods and how to arrange them in your day. Here I just want to give you a simple list of foods that you may want to put back into your diet. These slices of good news will be followed by two sections listing foods you may want to remove.

Foods to include that you may be avoiding:

Eggs
Eat the whole egg, including the yolk. You can even have more than two a day. Just be sure to eat good eggs from hormone-free, free-range chickens.

Meat
Whenever possible, choose meat from grass-fed, free-roaming and hormone-free animals. You don't even need to eat lean cuts. Animal fats can be very beneficial when your digestion is working properly. (If you are eating conventionally raised meats [meat from animals that are not grass-fed, hormone-free, free-roaming animals], it is important to consume lean cuts and avoid fat. Animals store their toxins in fat, like we do; so if an animal is pumped full of antibiotics and other harmful chemicals, you don't want to consume the animal's fat where much of those toxins will be stored.)

Fish
Try to find wild-caught options.

Butter
Real butter. Clarified butter and ghee are good options as well.

Extra virgin olive and coconut oils
Make sure they say "Raw" or "Extra Virgin" on the label.

Major Stay Aways

Most of the foods listed below will slow weight loss due to the big insulin spikes they often create or by the toxins they introduce into the body.

Sugar
You know this by now, right?

Artificial Sweeteners

Alcohol

Juice

Grains and grain-containing foods (like bread, cereal and baked treats)
Whole grain is not healthy like mainstream media tells you. It will still spike your insulin level and most whole grain breads are processed in a manner that removes anything nutritious and just leaves in the carbs.

Pasta

Rice
Brown rice is not great either and will spike insulin levels.

Potatoes in all forms
(A sweet potato is not a potato.)

Corn
Corn is a very difficult crop to grow successfully without jacking that crop up with chemicals. Therefore, when you consume corn, you are likely ingesting those chemicals. It is very hard to find a clean source of corn these days. Not to mention that there are likely only seventeen products manufactured today that do not contain corn and one of those products is a Toyota Camry. It's possible that I'm exaggerating, but probably not by much. Due to the fact that so many products contain

this chemical-ridden corn, I figure I'm consuming enough of this garbage by accident so I generally avoid corn when I'm given the option.

Pork
Eating pork freaks me out because there are laws in America specifying that if table scraps are fed to pigs behind a restaurant, the scraps must be boiled before being fed to the hogs. These laws were put into effect because, if a person eating at the restaurant has typhoid fever and scraps from his plate are not purified by boiling, it is possible to pass that typhoid fever through the hog eating those scraps. Hogs are referred to as an "unclean animal;" maybe that's because their digestive system does not sufficiently clean what they eat before it goes into their flesh.

Margarine or butter-replacement spreads
These products are often one molecule away from being plastic. If you leave them out overnight, bugs won't even eat them. Take the hint. They are not a healthy choice like advertisers would have you believe.

You May Or May Not Need To Avoid

Dairy
I find that most individuals will do well with butter (unless they have a strong Anabolic Imbalance). When it comes to other dairy products, it all depends on how well you can process those dairy proteins. Many lactose intolerant people can add a digestive enzyme supplement and consume dairy products once again. Others may need to avoid dairy altogether. In the next chapter I list specific dairy products that should be avoided or implemented depending on the specific imbalance. Beyond these uses, I have come across individuals who have a hard time losing weight as long as they are consuming dairy. They just can't process it correctly. If you see plateaus with your progress, try removing or reducing dairy and see if that speeds things up.

Soy
I view soy much in the same manner I do dairy. Some folks do okay eating soy. My advice is to generally limit soy if you feel like you need to include it. Soy has the ability to mimic estrogen in the body and can cause some freaky hormonal reactions in some people. This can be a big problem for vegans or vegetarians if they rely too heavily on soy for their

protein intake. Most people process fermented soy foods better than unfermented varieties.

Wha'd He Say?

In this chapter, you learned:

- Meat can be healthy if it is from hormone-free, grass-fed, free-range sources and if you can digest it properly.
- By eating vegan or vegetarian, you may be denying your body nutrients it requires.
- Organic foods are normally a better choice, but organic does not mean healthy. You still need to make good choices.
- Frozen organic produce can contain more nutrients than fresh organic produce.
- Margarine and butter-replacement spreads are not food and should not be consumed by any human.

CHAPTER FOURTEEN

Foods Specific To You

The search for a diet that works for everyone can stop now. Really. Shut it down. It's not gonna happen. You're better off wasting your time looking for a chocolate fountain of youth. Wasn't it Ponce De Leon himself who once said, "I hate this diet and I have yet to lose a single pound." Look at it realistically—if one diet worked for everybody, why are there so many diets?

As soon as you adopt a new base understanding that there is no diet that is right for every person, and there is no supplement that is right for every person, then you can stop throwing your time in the garbage looking for the magic diet or the "silver bullet." There are foods and supplements that can bring about changes in your body that will make you feel as if they have a magical effect, but they won't bring about the same results for your sister or even for your neighbor. Since these foods and supplements don't work for everyone, they're really not magic are they? They are just the more ideal choice for you and your chemistry.

Diet Is Determined By Strength Of Digestion

Instead of selecting your diet from the last magazine article you read, you might want to try eating according to what your digestion can handle. Yes, the goal is to correct digestive issues so you can broaden your selection. However, while you're improving your digestion, try adjusting your food selection according to your ability to digest.

If your HCL production appears to be low, proteins may be harder to digest. If your bile is not flowing properly, fats can be difficult to emulsify and process. If you've become insulin resistant or have a strong

Fat Burner Imbalance, you can have a hard time correctly processing carbohydrates and you may want to reduce the amount of starches you are eating. Understanding your current situation can help you better gauge what type of foods you should avoid and what foods you should eat.

Foods That Could Help

I really like the idea of using food choices to improve imbalances. Hippocrates said, "Let your food be your medicine and your medicine be your food." Seeing how Hippocrates is considered to be the "father of western medicine," I'm pretty sure western medicine stopped listening to Daddy at some point. It seems you would have a real hard time finding a medical doctor who would give you any advice about food at all. It's true some doctors are given a poster of a food pyramid and you can even look at it on the wall while your doctor fills out your prescriptions. I have clients with Type II Diabetes who tell me that their doctors never mentioned food to them. Even with Type II Diabetes our doctors don't seem to be teaching their patients that sugars and starches have the ability to quickly raise blood sugar levels that are already too high, as levels often are in diabetics. (By the way, I love that the Hippocratic Oath is to "do no harm." Do you really want someone working on you who's trying to "do no harm?" How about someone who's trying to do some good?)

Food (or nonfood in many cases) is what fuels our bodies. If you don't think the type of fuel you eat matters, try putting anything in the gas tank of your car other than what was intended to go there: Gas. If you really don't believe me, fill your car's gas tank with Gatorade or soda or Oreo cookies and then drive back to the bookstore so you can return this book. If you make it to the store, you're right. If not, you can read the rest of this book while you wait for AAA to pick you up. Just don't get upset if the tow truck driver wants to take a picture of you so he can show all his friends the person who crammed cookies into the gas tank. We really are smarter than this as a civilization. When we think about it, it's obvious: The type of food we eat matters. It's just very hard for us to see this concept when we have been taught so many misleading theories our whole lives. At least we now have the ability to open our eyes, if only a little.

Below I list food choices that can affect specific imbalances. For each imbalance, I list foods that seem to commonly improve that imbalance and other foods that appear to most frequently push a person further into that imbalance. Keep in mind that you are still an individual and foods that commonly push an imbalance one direction for most people may have an opposite reaction with you. That is why it is so important for you to monitor what you're doing and how your chemistry is moving. Because different individuals have different digestive predispositions and capacities, the same food can have a different effect on similar imbalances from person to person.

It's a lot of fun finding specific foods that can make you feel better, but most people cannot count on food alone. In nearly every case of a severe imbalance, those people's chemistries have been moving further out of balance for years or even decades. They have likely been making less than ideal choices for a long, long time. To push that chemistry back into balance, it's reasonable to think that they would have to make the right food choices for just as long, if their goal was to become balanced. That is not a scientific formula so don't hold too much weight in what I just said. It's just a good analogy so calm down and don't try to pull out a calendar to figure out the exact day in your life when you began to eat poorly. The point I'm trying to get across is that sometimes it will take more than food alone to straighten out a severe imbalance. But in most cases, eating foods that benefit an imbalance can reduce the required effort in other areas (like supplementation) so that you can reach your goals faster.

Supplements are a much more concentrated form of specific nutrients than what can be found in most foods. Some supplements are even made of what are called "complete foods" or "whole foods." No, not from the store, Whole Foods. These phrases just mean that these supplements are made from food instead of from a synthetic, fractionated form of that nutrient. I talk more about these supplements in chapter sixteen. I like to see people use supplements along with the correct food choices in order to see results faster, and then gradually reduce the amount of supplements they need until they can keep their body balanced with food choices alone. With that goal in mind, I spend this chapter digging into the foods that can be beneficial for each imbalance.

My final note about this chapter goes like this: If you have a severe imbalance that may be contributing to weight gain, and you see a food listed under an "avoid" column for that imbalance, that doesn't mean you can never eat that food again. You can eat that food tomorrow if you want—you'll just be slowing down your results. For example, soft-boiled eggs normally have the ability to push a person more anabolic. If you have a severe Anabolic Imbalance, the best plan is to avoid soft-boiled eggs until you become more balanced. But maybe you have a requirement in your life that makes it impossible to avoid soft-boiled eggs. If, for any reason, you feel you still need to eat soft-boiled eggs, you can try to increase your anti-anabolic protocol in other areas to allow you to eat a food that is going to push you the wrong direction (more anabolic). Maybe you need to really increase your food intake that will push you less anabolic. Maybe you can add another supplement to make up for it.

It is optimal to avoid the foods that will make a severe imbalance worse, but you do have options. You can get creative if you feel as though removing a food is not an option for you. You will learn that even the time of day that a food or supplement is implemented matters. This may allow you to keep some of your favorite foods in the mix by simply adjusting what time of the day you eat them.

Contradictions From Imbalance To Imbalance

You may notice that if you are dealing with more than one imbalance, "foods to implement" and "foods to avoid" may contradict each other from imbalance to imbalance. For example, foods that are recommended to help an Anabolic Imbalance may also be recommended to avoid for an Electrolyte Deficiency Imbalance. If you come across a similar circumstance, you may need to see what works best for you by watching your self-test numbers when you eat these foods.

Some of you are going to take the suggestions below and turn them into "rules" rather than suggestions based on principles. Please do not allow me to be more than a friend offering suggestions to think about.

You really only need to read about the foods below that are listed under the imbalances that showed up on your *Imbalance Guide*. You can skip the rest. I don't mind if you want to read about the foods that benefit each imbalance, just don't confuse yourself by soaking in information that does not apply to you and your chemistry. I am hoping that you've already performed your self-tests and know which imbalances you are dealing with so you can at least understand which imbalances to focus on the most. If you have not run your self-tests, is it because you hate me? Run your self-tests already.

Imbalance - Electrolyte Deficiency

Avoid
- Avoid drinking too much water or being unconscious about water intake

This doesn't mean you don't need more water, you may. However, you need to qualify to drink more water. If you have a low amount of minerals in the system, drinking a lot of water will just wash away the small amount you do have. Work on correcting digestion and increasing your unrefined salt intake and then you can increase your water as your blood pressure comes up.

- Avoid drinking distilled water or tap water

Since distilled water contains no minerals, drinking it can wash minerals out without replenishing them. Chlorine and fluoride in tap water can also reduce minerals in the body since the body needs to use those minerals to help safely remove the chlorine and fluoride from the body.

- Avoid eating too many sugars and especially starchy carbohydrates

These foods can spike insulin levels and cause your blood sugar to drop too low, too quickly.

Implement
- Correctly digesting your food
- Eating food

This means eating breakfast. Often because digestion is not functioning properly, understandably, many people skip breakfast. After all, why eat protein for breakfast when it's going to make you feel miserable for the next six hours? But if the mineral level is low because of poor digestion, as digestion is repaired, something needs to be given to the body to digest. Once the body sees that it has the ability to pull nutrients out of the food you're eating, the body is going to want more of that.

- Tomatoes and/or tomato sauce

Tomatoes have the ability to thicken your blood, thereby raising your blood pressure. If you like tomato sauce, using it is a great way to make just about any meal beneficial for an Electrolyte Deficiency Imbalance.

- Using an unrefined salt with your food

In my opinion, when it comes to food, unrefined salt can be the most important component to implement for an Electrolyte Deficiency Imbalance. Yes, it is true that correcting any digestive issues takes center stage for this imbalance. However, if you're not getting enough chloride into your system, your body can't begin to make its own HCL in the stomach. This is often the missing factor when a person has digestive issues.

When I have clients with extremely low blood pressure and all the numbers are pointing to a severe Electrolyte Deficiency Imbalance, I like to see them load up the unrefined salt at every meal as much as they can. I tell them that if they are eating lunch with a friend, the goal should be to use so much salt that their friend cries out, "What the heck is wrong with you?"

Obviously, you don't want to make your food gross. Don't add so much salt that you can't get through your meal without gagging. But if you can add salt to your meal, take a bite and it still tastes okay, you might want to add a little more. Just stop before it begins to taste like a salt lick. If you don't know what a salt lick is, google "salt lick" or "mineral lick." You will be intrigued by what you find. People use salt licks with horses a lot. It's kind of funny to see that many horse owners don't really understand why they give it to their horses. They just hear that it's beneficial so they do it. Nature photographers use a salt lick to attract wildlife. Animals will come from far and wide to load up on needed minerals. Yet, we humans still view salt as if it's a bad thing. Oops.

The word salary even comes from "salt." In Roman times, soldiers were paid in salt. Would you go to work every day and fight for your life if you were being paid in salt? Maybe you should. Maybe your life would be better since you would probably use some of that salt.

I'm not positive, but I believe it was Mother Theresa who once said, "Salt 'em if ya got 'em."

Imbalance - Electrolyte Excess

Avoid
- Avoid drinking tap water that is loaded with chlorine and/or fluoride

You may notice that I recommend avoiding some of the same things for opposite imbalances. For example, I've listed avoiding tap water under Electrolyte Deficiency as well as Electrolyte Excess. Logic might tell you that if an item is bad for one imbalance, it should be good for the opposite imbalance. However, that is not always the case. It can sometimes be beneficial to avoid a specific item from imbalance to imbalance, and for totally different reasons.

For an Electrolyte Deficiency Imbalance, it was recommended to avoid tap water containing chlorine or fluoride because drinking this water can strip the body of needed minerals. With an Electrolyte Excess Imbalance, tap water should also be avoided but for different reasons. If the body's waste removal systems are not working optimally, chemicals from the tap water can build up, making the bloodstream thicker and harder to keep clean. Remember, with an Electrolyte Excess Imbalance, the blood is often too thick so it doesn't help to bring in more filth and muddy up the system. Drinking adequate water is fundamental in helping the kidneys. In this regard, intake of clean water can equate to changing the bag in the vacuum cleaners of the blood.

- Avoid eating too many sugars or starchy carbohydrates

Sugars and carbohydrates can thicken the blood; therefore, excessive consumption is not recommended with an Electrolyte Excess Imbalance. Measuring blood sugar with a glucometer can be helpful.

- Avoid taking antacids

Antacids restrict proper digestion. Undigested foods become a waste product that the body has to deal with.

- Avoid eating polyunsaturated oils

This can include some salad dressings, margarine, mayonnaise and foods fried or cooked with vegetable oils. Coconut oil, real butter and unheated virgin olive oil are all okay.

<u>Implement</u>
- Using an unrefined salt with your food

The initial thought for someone with an Electrolyte Excess Imbalance would be to avoid salt. It is true that if you add salt with this imbalance, you will want to monitor your blood pressure and make sure it does not go up. However, if adding unrefined salt can provide the body with the chloride needed to improve HCL production, higher HCL production can improve digestion, therefore, reducing the junk in the system that was created as a result of improper digestion. Now, the body has one less burden and can focus on removing waste. This can help the body reduce blood pressure.

- Correcting any digestive issues so you can properly break down your food
- Drinking more water
- Eating a lot of low-starch green vegetables

Imbalance - Anabolic

<u>Avoid</u>
- Avoid foods made with hydrogenated and polyunsaturated fatty acids: Canola, corn and soy oils
- Avoid ice cream
- Avoid butter
- Avoid cream
- Avoid cheese
- Avoid juices
- Avoid foods made with sugar
- Avoid coffee
- Avoid tea
- Avoid soda
- Avoid excessive fruit
- Avoid vinegar
- Avoid poached or soft-boiled eggs

<u>Implement</u>
- Non-starchy vegetables
- Fish (especially salmon)
- Unheated virgin olive oil
- Flax seed oil (in a pearl-type gel cap is best; do not heat flax seed oil)
- Ground flax seed (fresh ground whole seed)
- Lemon juice

- Citrus fruit
- Sardines
- Fried or omelet-style eggs in the morning (not Egg-Beaters or egg whites)

Even in a time crunch, if you make hard-boiled eggs, you can keep them in the fridge and grab one on the run in the morning. When your digestion is working correctly, a hard-boiled or hard-cooked egg can be a powerful anti-anabolic meal and can even reduce your need for anti-anabolic supplements.

Powerful Anti-Anabolic Meal

There is a widely used recipe from the Budwig Diet that I feel to be very anti-anabolic inducing. It's basically cottage cheese and flax seed oil blended together with ground flax seed stirred in, but there are specifics that you have to follow for the science to work.

The reasons this recipe works are: First, it contains all the fatty acids to help push a person less anabolic, and second, when the sulfur proteins in the cottage cheese are blended at the molecular level with the fatty acids, a sulfur compound is created that can get into the cells where needed. Sulfur is a very strong anti-anabolic substance.

This is the recipe:
1. Take 3 Tbs of extra virgin olive oil. (The Budwig Diet calls for cold-pressed flax seed oil, but it appears that most flax seed oil sold in stores is rancid before it leaves the shelves. Freshly made flax seed oil would be acceptable, but it can be hard to find. The extra virgin olive oil is an excellent replacement.)
2. Blend with 6 Tbs of cottage cheese. Stirring them together will not work. They need to be blended so that the molecules join together. An immersion blender is the best way to do that because one serving is too small to put in a blender or food processor. One of those hand held, single-blade immersion blenders is best, but a juice blender will do too. Blend the first two ingredients for about a minute. It will look like pudding.
3. Grind 2 Tbs of fresh flax seeds (a coffee grinder works well and will probably cost you about $30). It's important to grind them fresh because the lignans will lose their effectiveness after about 30 minutes. For this reason, the ground flax seed from the store does not work the same. Once ground, just stir it into the cottage cheese mixture with a spoon.
4. Optional: Add broken up walnuts or Brazil nuts. Make sure they are raw and not roasted.

If you're super anabolic, eating this whenever you have time may be beneficial, but earlier in the day is more optimal than at night since people are meant to be more catabolic during the day. Therefore, this dish is best eaten at breakfast or as a snack before lunch.

Imbalance - Catabolic

Avoid

- Avoid flax seed oil
- Avoid fish oils
- Avoid DHEA (a popular supplement)
- Avoid fried foods
- Avoid canned or processed meats and fish
- Avoid foods made with hydrogenated and polyunsaturated fatty acids: Canola, corn and soy oils
- If you eat fried or hard-boiled eggs, eat them only in the morning and limit them

Implement

- Poached or soft-boiled eggs, especially at night
- Non-starchy vegetables
- Real butter/cream/whipped cream (especially in the evening)
- Fresh cheeses such as cottage, mozzarella, and cream cheese (these are not aged cheeses)
- Coconut oil (or use my coconut yummy recipe found in chapter ten)

Imbalance - Carb Burner

Avoid

- Avoid sugar and similar items like corn syrup and honey
- Avoid fruit juices and large quantities of fruit
- Avoid coffee, tea, and alcohol
- Avoid eating polyunsaturated oils

This can include some salad dressings, margarine, mayonnaise and foods fried or cooked with vegetable oils. Coconut oil, real butter and unheated virgin olive oil are all okay.

- Avoid meals consisting predominantly of sugars or starches

It could be beneficial for you to include at least a small serving of protein and appropriate fats in each meal.

Implement
- Eating non-starch vegetables
- Vegetables like zucchini, squash, broccoli and asparagus may be beneficial because they can provide carbs without such a high level of carbs that the meal spikes your insulin levels.
- Eating some carbs early in the day, but try to avoid meals made up predominantly of carbs.
- Keeping your glucometer on you at all times
- Knowing when your blood sugar is low (say, below 70) will allow you to manage your blood sugar instead of being at the mercy of it.

Imbalance - Fat Burner

While you are improving this imbalance, it is important to reduce your starch and sugar intake. (Keep in mind that if you experience drops in your blood sugar and you need starches or sugars from time to time in order to continue functioning, small amounts of sugar will often bring a better result than starches will. But for most people with this imbalance, limiting intake of both starches and sugars will be beneficial.) When you reduce one type of nutrient, another type must be increased to fill in the gaps. I like to increase fat intake with this imbalance since the body appears to be burning fat well. However, it is important that bile is flowing properly so you can emulsify those fats. If you increase fat intake, and bile is not flowing well, it could result in weight gain or breakouts caused by the body trying to push fats that have not been emulsified out of the body through the skin.

Avoid
- Avoid sugar and similar items like corn syrup and honey
- Avoid fruit juices and large quantities of fruit
- Avoid drinking alcohol and soda
- Avoid eating polyunsaturated oils
- This can include some salad dressings, margarine, mayonnaise and foods fried or cooked with vegetable oils. Coconut oil, real butter and unheated virgin olive oil are all okay.
- Avoid meals consisting predominantly of sugars or starches
- It could be beneficial for you to include at least a small serving of protein and appropriate fats in each meal.

Implement
- Consuming appropriate fats

- These can include coconut oil, real butter, unheated virgin olive oil, and those found in eggs (the whole egg) or animal proteins.
- Keep your glucometer on you for measuring when your blood sugar is high or low. This will allow you to manage blood sugar instead of being at the mercy of it.

Wha'd He Say?

In this chapter, you learned:

- The diet that is right for you should be determined by your ability to digest and process different types of nutrients.
- The lists in this chapter do not provide you with the only foods you are allowed to eat. If you are experiencing a specific imbalance, eating the foods in the "Implement" list as often as you can, may improve that imbalance. Including other foods in your diet, however, is appropriate and beneficial.
- If your favorite food is listed under "Avoid" for an imbalance you are experiencing, that does not mean you can never eat that food again. Once you take the steps to improve that imbalance, you should be able to enjoy that food again in moderation.

CHAPTER FIFTEEN

Meal Planning

Before I get into meal planning, I first want to review four general guidelines you'll need to keep in mind while putting together your weight loss plan.

Weight Loss Guidelines

1. You must, must, must, must fix any aspects of digestion that are not working optimally.
2. Give your body the minerals and nutrients it needs so you can quiet your cravings. If you're dealing with cravings, how are you going to stick to a plan? You can reduce cravings by correcting digestion, eating more nutrient rich foods, utilizing an unrefined salt, and/or using the right supplements.
3. Reduce starches, carbs, sugars and alcohol at key times in order to allow insulin levels to come down (you must first qualify to do this by raising mineral levels if yours are low).
4. Improve any imbalances that are restricting weight loss.

Following those main guidelines can put you on the right path to weight loss. Remember, just checking off one item from that list may not help you very much. That would be like going on a deep sea fishing trip and only making sure you have your life vest. A life vest is important, but how many fish are you going to catch if you don't have a boat, fishing gear, bait, and one of those hats that make every human look like an eighty-year-old man? You need to make sure all of these guidelines are covered.

Avoid Boredom

When you cut out processed junk and include more real food, until you learn how to get creative, you may be eating a lot of the same foods every day—a lot of eggs, chicken and green vegetables. Once a week, take some time to find new recipes and provide yourself with variety in your meals. I produce a web series you can find at www.CookForYourChemistry.com. There, you'll even find recipes geared toward improving specific imbalances. You can find more free recipes at www.DoneWithThatBooks.com and if you register with *The Coalition*, there are loads on that site as well.

To get you started, here are a few ideas on how to put a little variety into those healthy staples without having to follow a recipe.

Prepare
Pick a day, once a week, to be your cooking day. You may prefer to cook twice a week and prepare less each time. Then, simply get yourself set up for the week. Most people fail to lose weight because they wait until they're already starving to figure out what they're going to eat next. How often do you make good choices while you're hungry enough to eat a squirrel if it would just hold still for a minute? Know what you're going to eat at your next meal before it's time to eat that meal and you will have much greater success.

- Bake enough chicken to last five to seven days at a time.
- Get a salad spinner, then wash and shred enough lettuce for the week. It stays crisp in the spinner for five to seven days and you always have a salad ready to go. You can grab a handful, cut up a chicken breast that you already baked and you have a salad in two minutes.
- Bake or roast mixed vegetables that you can keep in the fridge. Heat them up with a chicken breast for an easy lunch.
- Buy a convection toaster oven for about $100. You can pop in any pre-cooked food and it will heat up in ten minutes. I explain microwaves in chapter eighteen and why you won't want to use them anymore.

Eggs
Eggs truly are the perfect food. Now that you've moved past the cholesterol and dietary fat fiction that was scaring you away from eggs,

including them on a regular basis can be a great way to speed up weight loss.

- Use leftover veggies in an omelet or scramble the next morning. Have them cooked, and ready to cut up and add to an egg dish. If you have to cook the veggies and then add them to your eggs, you'll tell yourself you don't have time and end up grabbing a muffin at the gas station.
- Mix a variety of veggies into your eggs. Make it different every time. You can even cut up some of the chicken you baked the day before and mix that into your omelet or scramble too. People often freak out when I say that, like you're not allowed to mix chicken into eggs since eggs become chickens or something. Get over yourself and mix it in. It's so good and gives the eggs a totally different flavor. If you stick with eating plain eggs, you will last maybe two weeks before you'll be tired of them. Mix it up.
- Keep hard boiled eggs on hand for a great on-the-go meal or snack.

Chicken

Chicken breast can get pretty boring if you're eating it every day. However, if you mix up the type of chicken you're eating, how it's prepared and what you eat it with, it can be new and exciting every time. Does this take effort? You bet it does. Carrying an extra hundred pounds up the stairs takes effort too. Know that doing it the easy way is how you got to where you are now. Doing it the right way is how you're going to get to where you want to be.

- Try new seasonings. Baking is the easiest way to prepare chicken, in my opinion. Try sprinkling on new seasonings until you find four or five flavors you really like. Most seasonings are okay. I like the pre-mixed varieties you can find at most grocery stores like italian seasonings, poultry seasonings, garlic mixtures or simply salt and pepper can be a great combo.
- Stir frys are quick and easy. By adding a tablespoon of coconut oil to a pan, tossing in a raw, cut-up chicken breast, you now have a base for any type of stir fry. Add different veggies every time until you find your favorite mixtures. If you have an Electrolyte Deficiency Imbalance, this is also a great time to mix in a half teaspoon of blackstrap molasses to boost the mineral levels in your meal. (Yes, I understand that sounds a little freaky but you don't really taste it if you use other seasonings too. Just remember that the molasses does contain sugars, so use it only if you need the mineral lift.)
- If you're tired of chicken breast, try chicken legs, thighs, or cook a whole chicken. If you're eating clean, hormone-free, free-range

chicken, you don't need to stick to only the lean breast meat. Mix it up. Ground chicken or turkey is a great way to add variety as well.

- Make sauces or use low-carb dressings to flavor meals. In a refrigerated section of most health food stores, you can find low-carb dressings containing no added sugar. Look for varieties made predominantly of olive oil, when possible. Higher fat content is okay as long as sugars are low.

Veggies

Steamed vegetables are a healthy choice, but that doesn't mean that's the only way you're allowed to eat your veggies. Finding ways to change the way you're preparing your greens can keep you interested enough to continue eating them.

- People often get tired of having vegetables steamed and plain. That's advanced healthy eating and I don't expect you to jump right into a ninja move like that. Remember that you need healthy fats; and while most veggies don't contain fats, they are the perfect food to dump more fats onto and into your mouth. If you're experiencing a Catabolic Imbalance or if you are balanced, butter can be an excellent healthy fat to be added to all your cooked veggies. If you have an Anabolic Imbalance, take steps to improve that imbalance and you will be able to use butter in moderation as well.
- When not steaming, try to cook your veggies in coconut oil. Adding olive oil to veggies after they are cooked can be excellent variety and a good way to include more fats. However, cooking in olive oil is not as beneficial as cooking in coconut oil, as some believe that cooking olive oil can change how those fats react in the body.
- Stir frys are the easiest way to change how your veggies taste. You can not only change the veggies you are cooking, you can also change the herbs and seasonings you are mixing into your stir fry.
- If you cook enough servings to last for a few days, you can heat them up in your convection toaster oven and they will taste just as good as when you first cooked them.

Building A Meal

The foundation of every meal should start with protein (animal protein being the optimal choice). You will likely eat more veggies than protein in each meal, but I still like to view the protein as the starting point. You also want to include appropriate fats and a vegetable source in as many meals as possible. For those who need to include medium-carb foods because your mineral content is too low, try to eat those carbs with protein. A snack of fruit is okay to eat alone; but with most other medium-carb foods, try to eat them with protein.

I don't want you to weigh your food or use a protractor to measure the circumference of a serving of broccoli or anything complicated like that. That takes way too much time and I'm hoping you create a life for yourself in your new skinny jeans. Instead, just listen to your body and use your hand to estimate serving sizes. For breakfast, lunch and dinner, your protein serving should equate to about the size of your palm, both in size and thickness. Your vegetable serving should be about the size of your whole hand. Use that gauge as a starting point and then listen to your body. If you start to feel full, don't keep cramming food down your gullet. An oversized healthy meal can spike insulin levels in the same way carbs or sugars can.

Once you have digestion working correctly, and you're giving your body healthy proteins, fats and low-starch carbohydrates at every meal, you will feel satiated after most meals. If you still feel hungry, you may need to increase your servings. The more likely scenario is that you need to increase your healthy fat intake. Consuming plenty of appropriate fats is a great way to insure feeling satisfied after a meal.

Planning A Day

Knowing everything you're going to eat the following day is an excellent way to succeed. The better you plan, the more effortless your weight loss will seem. Maybe you don't know exactly what you're going to eat for lunch, but you know the restaurant you're going to and you know they have five or six choices that work for you.

In this chapter I include sample meal plans that show my idea for an optimal day of eating. Visit www.DoneWithThatBooks.com for many more sample meal plans. You will even find plans tailored to specific imbalances and all of this information is available to you for free. You can take all the thinking out of your meal planning by simply using exactly what I've laid out. I prefer to see you use the sample plans for a month or two while you learn to create your own. By learning how to create your own, you become totally independent and in charge of your nutrition.

Planning a Week

If you use the meal plans I've posted on www.DoneWithThatBooks.com, you can select an entire week and download the shopping list for that week. Keep in mind that the initial shopping trips may be a little more expensive as you load up on different seasonings and such. However, once you have those in your pantry, future shopping trips can be more affordable.

This system can be like training wheels that allow you to teach yourself how to cook your own healthy meals. Not only will this save you a lot of cash; if you cook for someone on a date, you may actually get a follow-up date. With every online meal plan, if you don't know how to make a dish, you can simply click on the name and the recipe and instructions will appear before you. I'm not magic, it's just a website.

If you use the cooking day I described earlier in this chapter, you can really reduce prep time for most meals. Otherwise, if you have to spend thirty minutes preparing each meal each day, it will be harder for you to keep up this lifestyle. Make it easy for yourself while you're adjusting your skills from speaking clearly in the drive-through intercom to creating nutritious and delicious food for yourself.

If you use meal plans designed to help improve a specific imbalance, you must continue monitoring yourself every week or so. If your chemistry begins to be more balanced, be sure to adjust your food intake as well. Include more meals geared toward a balanced chemistry so you don't create an imbalance in the other direction.

Sample Meal Plans

Here are a few sample plans that, if your digestion is working well, will keep you feeling satiated and set you up for some great weight loss. The Coconut Yummies listed below are from the recipe in chapter ten.

Sample Balanced Meal Plan

Breakfast
3-egg scramble cooked in coconut oil with spinach, broccoli and ¼ of a sliced chicken breast
1 Tbs butter on top
Snack (approx. 3 hours later)
Celery stalks with almond butter
Lunch
Salad with grilled chicken, half an avocado, sprouts and a low-carb, full-fat olive oil based dressing
1 Coconut Yummy
Snack (approx. 3 hours later)
Chocolate egg-white protein shake (I like Jay Robb and MRM brands): 1.5 scoops of protein powder, water, ice, and handful of kale or spinach
Dinner (approx. 3 hours later)
Steak with asparagus
1 Coconut Yummy

Sample Meal Plan Including Medium-Carbs

Breakfast
3-egg scramble cooked in coconut oil with peppers and onions
1 Tbs butter on top
Snack (approx. 3 hours later)
Handful of berries
Lunch
Grilled chicken, avocado and a low-carb garlic dressing served with a half cup of kidney beans
1 Coconut Yummy
Snack (approx. 3 hours later)
Chocolate egg-white protein shake (I like Jay Robb and MRM brands): 1.5 scoops of protein powder, water, ice, and handful of kale or spinach
Dinner (approx. 3 hours later)
Grilled chicken with carrots and broccoli
1 Tbs butter on top
1 Coconut Yummy

Sample Pro-Anabolic Meal Plan

This is a meal plan that could be used by people with a Catabolic Imbalance who wish to push their chemistry more anabolic.

Breakfast
3-egg omelet cooked in coconut oil with spinach
1 Tbs butter on top
1 Coconut Yummy
Snack (approx. 3 hours later)
Broccoli and cucumbers with hummus
Lunch
2 baked chicken legs with stir fried zucchini, squash and sugar snap peas cooked in coconut oil and with basil cream sauce on top
1 Coconut Yummy
Snack (approx. 3 hours later)
Chocolate egg-white protein shake (I like Jay Robb and MRM brands): 1.5 scoops of protein powder, water, ice, and handful of kale or spinach
Dinner (approx. 3 hours later)
3 poached eggs with a side of steamed broccoli
1 Tbs butter on top
1 Coconut Yummy

Sample Pro-Catabolic Meal Plan

This is a meal plan that could be used by people with an Anabolic Imbalance who wish to push their chemistry more catabolic.

Breakfast
2 hard-boiled eggs dipped in extra virgin olive oil, unrefined salt and pepper
Snack (approx. 3 hours later)
Handful of raw almonds
Lunch
Grilled salmon salad with avocado, extra virgin olive oil and italian herbs
Snack (approx. 3 hours later)
Chocolate egg-white protein shake (I like Jay Robb and MRM brands): 1.5 scoops of protein powder, water, ice, and handful of kale or spinach.
Dinner (approx. 3 hours later)

2 baked chicken legs with a side of broccoli and leeks, sautéed in coconut oil, sprinkled with extra virgin olive oil and herbs (after cooking)

Meal Plans For Imbalances

While browsing meal plans at www.DoneWithThatBooks.com, you'll see that I split meal plans into four categories: Balanced Plans, Medium-Carb Plans, Pro-Anabolic Plans, and Pro-Catabolic Plans. Here are few notes for using these plans with specific imbalances.

Electrolyte Deficiency/Excess Imbalances

I don't provide any plans designed to benefit those dealing with electrolyte imbalances because most of your efforts to improve these imbalances will come in the form of improving digestion, adding unrefined salt or other supplemented mineral lifters, or adjusting your water intake.

Anabolic/Catabolic Imbalances

If an Anabolic or Catabolic Imbalance showed up on your *Imbalance Guide*, using these designed meal plans can sometimes be enough to push an individual in the right direction. If your imbalance appears to be strong, feel free to include as many as you like of these meal plans designed for your imbalance. You must, however, keep an eye on your chemistry so you can adjust your meals once you appear more balanced.

Fat Burner and Carb Burner Imbalances

If a Carb Burner Imbalance showed up on your *Imbalance Guide*, you may want to include some meals from the Medium-Carb Plans. These menus will provide you with the carbs your body needs while you improve digestion, adjust imbalanced pHs, and teach your body how to use fat for fuel instead of predominantly burning carbohydrates. As this imbalance improves, reducing the number of medium-carb meals you eat may increase your weight-loss efforts. If you start to go nuts or your cravings go crazy, increase the number of medium-carb meals you eat until you have raised your mineral levels.

If a Fat Burner Imbalance showed up on your Imbalance Guide, choosing from the balanced menus, or selecting meals that may improve an Anabolic or Catabolic Imbalance you are dealing with, could be appropriate for you. All of these meals are geared toward weight loss and are, therefore, appropriate for a Fat Burner Imbalance.

Wha'd He Say?

In this chapter, you learned:

- Before you worry about what foods to eat, be sure you are tackling the four weight loss guidelines described in this chapter.
- Cook enough extra food to last four to seven days, allowing you to quickly heat up meals.
- Find meal plans specific to your imbalances, shopping lists and recipes at www.DoneWithThatBooks.com.
- If you are using meal plans designed to improve an imbalance, be sure to monitor your chemistry so you know when to make adjustments with your food choices.

CHAPTER SIXTEEN

Supplements That Could Help

It seems we are always hearing something good or bad about supplements in the news or in health magazines. The truth is that the media is all correct in some way or another—all the good and all the bad. Since every person is different and is experiencing different imbalances, specific supplements can either correct that person's imbalance or exacerbate it. Beyond the fact that we need to use the right supplements that will benefit our biological individuality, we also need to use supplements that the body can assimilate. Many supplements on the market today are not worth the bottle they're sold in. I'll teach you what to look for and where to get quality supplements that are right for you. Since many of you will need the aid of supplements in order to improve your digestion or imbalances that are restricting weight loss, don't take this information lightly. You don't want to waste your money on supplements that are not effective for you.

Many supplements that you can buy in the store are junk. What's worse is it appears that some products may even be made that way intentionally. Most vitamins, minerals and herbs have the ability to move body chemistry. The problem is that most consumers don't know anything about body chemistry and what vitamins will move that chemistry which direction. Wouldn't it make sense that if the vitamin manufacturers didn't want to deal with lawsuits all day long, they could just add binders to the supplements that make them very hard to assimilate?

Binders, lubricants and fillers are often added to supplements to hold tablets together, improve the ability of the supplements to run through the processing machinery faster and easier, or to make the supplements cheaper to manufacture. Any number of these added ingredients can reduce your body's ability to assimilate the nutrients found in those supplements. It is said that, with most consumer-based supplements, you can assimilate only between 4-12% of what's in them. In that way, it's difficult for people to push their chemistry the wrong way and there's no lawsuit. Whether companies are adding these binders to save money or to avoid lawsuits really doesn't matter. Either way, you still don't get an effective product.

There are companies that make high quality supplements without the harmful binders in them. The trick is that most of these companies sell their products only to qualified health care practitioners. In that way, if there's a lawsuit, it falls on the practitioner and not on the company. Di-calcium phosphate is a binder I like to try and avoid when buying supplements because it can restrict your ability to assimilate nutrients—not only from the supplement, but also from the food you're eating.

Most people choose a supplement because they read that it is good for a specific symptom. Little do they understand that a chemical imbalance is normally causing that symptom. If the supplement they choose can help correct that imbalance, they may see good results. If it doesn't, they will see bad results. Remember, one symptom can have many different underlying causes, so it is very common that two different people with the same symptom can experience very different results using the same supplement. Have I mentioned that it's not a good idea to treat your symptoms? If you don't wake up at least once in the middle of the night hearing me say, "Don't treat your symptoms," I will have failed in my efforts to teach you to look at your underlying causes measured using chemistry instead of looking at your symptoms. Since you now have a better idea of where your chemistry is, you have an edge that most people never get to experience. Welcome to where all the cool kids hang out.

Understand this: You're not going to be able to pop a few supplements and correct everything that's been going wrong for the past fifteen years. Supplements are not witchcraft. You're going to have to find a way to eliminate some of the things that are making these imbalances worse and add in new choices that will help you correct them. Any supplement usage is just a boost to help it happen quicker. None of the supplements I talk about in this book are intended to be used indefinitely like an over-the-counter drug often can be. These supplements are meant to correct deficiency or excess issues, and then a person should reduce what they're using until they don't need them anymore. Enzymes are the only exception, as I mentioned in chapter three. Again, when people start to work on their bodies, they may need to use a lot of supplements in the beginning to get things going in the right direction; then they will be able to reduce supplements as imbalances get corrected.

What If I Hate Taking Supplements?

No problem. You always have the option to continue being miserable (yes, I understand I'm annoying). The truth is, many people will be able to greatly improve their situation with food choices alone, or maybe just adding a good unrefined salt. I see that happen all the time. I also see people who are so screwed up, not only do they need the help of good supplements, they often need the help of a lot of them in the beginning.

Once you get in the habit of using supplements, it can be as easy as washing your hair. Yet, it's very interesting how averse some people are to using supplements at all. I have talked with people who have been suffering for years or even decades from issues like insomnia, constipation or diarrhea. They tell me that they don't like to put anything unknown in their body. That's okay. I can understand wanting to keep bad stuff out of your body. But with chronic issues like those mentioned, your body is screaming at you that things are not going as planned and it could really use some help. Take the time to learn more about supplements that could help you so you can feel good about using them.

I've already gone over why we hear so many good and bad stories about supplements. Yet, if you know which supplements are appropriate for you, and how to find the good ones, you're miles ahead of most people. Beyond all that, don't you think it's a little silly to avoid supplements because you're not sure what they're going to do to your body, yet you feel great about keeping candy bars in your desk that contain chemicals and artificial sweeteners that you *know* are harmful? It's up to you to make your own decisions. All I can do is point out how ridiculous some of your decisions are.

Don't view taking a lot of supplements as popping a bunch of pills. Many natural supplements are concentrated forms of specific nutrients, many made directly from food itself. So, you can view these supplements as part of your food. It's a much more convenient way to get the specific nutrients your body is looking for, rather than needing to shop at fifteen different farmer's markets to find a specific type of organic beet green. Who has time for that? If you view the supplements as the bane of your existence, you're obviously not going to feel good about taking them. A hatred for taking supplements could certainly reduce the benefits that those supplements could bring. However, if you view them as a convenient way to cheat and reach your goals faster, supplements can make your life a whole lot easier.

I can't recommend specific supplements to you, so don't waste your time emailing me questions about what you should be using. There are legal ramifications that don't allow me to help in that regard. But in this book, I can show you which supplements appear to help correct certain imbalances and I can even tell you what supplements I may take if I were trying to correct an imbalance. After you have that information you can decide for yourself if you want to try anything. Before I get into the supplements that can help improve specific imbalances, let me review the digestive supplements that seem to be beneficial for those who need to improve their digestion. When needed, these supplements will always be far more important than any other choices when it comes to weight loss.

Digestive Supplement Review

www.NaturalReference.com
Brand: Empirical Labs

Betaine HCL (See the HCL warning under *Improving Your Stomach Acid* in chapter three.)
1-5 per meal (In the middle of the meal.)

Beet Flow
2-3 per meal

Digesti-zyme
1-2 per meal

Fiber

Supplementing fiber is flat out cheating. At least you'll feel like you're cheating because results will show a lot faster. If all you do is supplement fiber, your results may not improve drastically. But if you're doing everything else correctly, adding a fiber supplement will give your results an excellent boost. It hardly matters whether you add a fiber powder to a shake, use fiber capsules or simply focus on more fiber in your diet. Ingesting more fiber is all that counts. I find that most people can use fiber capsules with the greatest level of consistency, because it's so easy. I like Fiber-Plex from Douglas Laboratories (available on www.NaturalReference.com) or Gastro Fiber from Standard Process. However, finding what floats your boat is the best way to go.

Improving Imbalances Through Supplementation

As I go through the imbalances, I list supplements that seem to be beneficial for each imbalance. Just be sure to understand that you are responsible for your own health and you have to decide what dosage is best for you. After you begin using a supplement, don't forget how important it is to continue to run your self-tests and monitor your numbers. Monitoring your numbers can help guide you in the dose you are using for many supplements, once you understand how a supplement can affect your body chemistry.

If you are currently working with healthcare professionals, you should always let them know what you are considering using just to make sure it is not contradicting anything they have you using already. Below, I'm not making any suggestions to you because I don't know you. You do remember that you only bought my book and we're not really talking, right? So, I couldn't possibly have a clue what your chemistry is or how much of each supplement you should take and when. I'm sure you see that would be a ridiculous assumption. I'm just listing supplements that I have seen people use with success.

I also list supplements that are contraindicated for each imbalance. This is very important because you don't want to try to fix one imbalance and simultaneously worsen another imbalance that showed up on your *Imbalance Guide*. For example, you may see that L-Glutamine can help a

Catabolic Imbalance so you decide to use it since your Catabolic Imbalance was so strong. But L-Glutamine is contraindicated for an Electrolyte Excess Imbalance, so if you also showed an Electrolyte Excess Imbalance, L-Glutamine could actually exacerbate that issue. Pay attention to what you're doing; and before you use a supplement to improve one imbalance, make sure it is not listed under the "avoid" section of another imbalance that showed up on your *Imbalance Guide*. This is one of the reasons why it can be so beneficial to employ the help of professional health coaches who understand these principles. Not only have they studied these principles extensively, they have also seen these fundamentals work, first hand, in their clients' efforts, so they can help you eliminate time-wasting moves.

For those of you working with a health coach, there will be a wider variety of more effective supplements available to you. Many of the higher quality supplements that are geared toward correcting the imbalances I talk about in this book are sold only through professionals. You'll need to find a health coach in your area if you feel you need to step up your game. Due to the fact that consumers can't purchase these supplements, I don't list them here.

The biggest mistake I see consumers make when it comes to supplements is that they will buy a supplement because their friend tells them it is good for a specific symptom—they'll start to use it and they will feel better. "Yay! I found something that works," they tell themselves. They will then continue to use this supplement FOREVER! No matter what. Even if the symptom comes back or gets worse, they will continue to use that supplement because they think, "Well, this helped me before so it must be something else that is causing the problem or the problem must just be escalating and now I need to add something else too." Don't do that. I've smacked people in the head for less than that. **Watch your numbers, see the patterns, and adjust what you're doing accordingly.** I can't emphasize that enough.

Before I get to the imbalances, my final point is this: Under some imbalances I list quite a few supplements that may help that imbalance. That does not mean that you should use all of those supplements just because that imbalance showed up on your *Imbalance Guide*. Unless your imbalance appears to be very strong, you might want to start with just one or two of the supplements listed under a given imbalance and then see if your self-testing numbers improve, indicating the imbalance is improving. If you don't see improvement, it might be time to add another supplement that is listed as beneficial under that imbalance.

Just pay attention to what you're doing and start slow and easy instead of throwing fifteen new supplements into your body at once.

My only exception to this slow-and-easy rule is if you are looking at digestive issues that need attention. When there are digestive issues, and it's likely there will be for most people dealing with weight gain, you need to address all aspects of digestion. Don't start by using just HCL and think you can add Beet Flow later. You need to address the lack of acid and use the Beet Flow to help bile flow correctly. You also need to make sure you are using some type of digestive enzyme to fully improve digestive issues. With this understanding, it's simple to see that the "start off slowly" approach does not apply to digestion. You still want to start off slowly with your *quantities* and build your way up; but when it comes to digestion, you really want to hit all the angles from the beginning.

Imbalance - Electrolyte Deficiency

The most important factors with an Electrolyte Deficiency Imbalance are correcting digestion and adding more unrefined salt. Try to make these your priorities and add other supplements from below as secondary tools.

Often Used With This Imbalance

- **L-Glutamine** An amino acid - Avoid with an Anabolic Imbalance. L-Glutamine can be bought in powder or capsule form in just about any health food store. It's a good idea to use powder since many people use doses of a full teaspoon at a time. You would need to take a lot of capsules to equal one teaspoon. If you become constipated while using L-Glutamine, you could be using too much and may need to reduce your dose.
- **L-Tyrosine** An amino acid - Avoid with a Catabolic Imbalance. (Avoid at night.)
- **Zinc** Keep the dose low with an Anabolic Imbalance.
- **Blackstrap Molasses**

- **Vitamin E**
- **L-Arginine** An amino acid.

Imbalance - Electrolyte Excess

Use water as a supplement. If you have an Electrolyte Excess Imbalance, odds are great that you are not drinking enough water. If you also have a Catabolic Imbalance, and if drinking more water gives you diarrhea, first improve your Catabolic Imbalance; and then you may be able to increase your water intake without inducing a loose stool.

Often Used With This Imbalance

- **L-Taurine** An amino acid - Avoid with a Catabolic Imbalance. (Best taken in the morning, and near lunch.)
- **Vitamin E** Avoid with an Anabolic or Carb Burner Imbalance. (Best taken with dinner.)

Avoid With This Imbalance

- **Vitamin D3**
- **L-Glutamine** An amino acid.

Imbalance - Anabolic

Often Used With This Imbalance

- **Vitamin B12** Can also help the body burn fat. (Best taken with breakfast and/or lunch. Avoid at night.)
- **Magnesium** (Best taken with breakfast and/or lunch. Avoid at night.)
- **Vitamin A** (Best taken with breakfast and/or lunch. Avoid at night.)
- **L-Tyrosine** An amino acid. (Avoid at night.)
- **Flax Seed Oil** Pearl form or gel cap is best. (Best taken with breakfast and/or lunch. Avoid at night.)

Avoid With This Imbalance

- **L-Glutamine** An amino acid.

- **L-Arginine** An amino acid.
- **Vitamin E**
- **Potassium Citrate**

Imbalance - Catabolic

Don't forget about poached or soft-boiled eggs with this imbalance. Any type of egg where the yolk is still runny can benefit a Catabolic Imbalance. Be sure to use hormone-free eggs. Real butter and coconut oil can also be considered to create supplement-like, beneficial results for some people with a Catabolic Imbalance.

Often Used With This Imbalance

- **L-Glutamine** An amino acid - Avoid with an Electrolyte Excess Imbalance. (Best taken after dinner, before bed, away from food.)
- **Vitamin E** Avoid with an Electrolyte Deficiency or Carb Burner Imbalance. (Best taken with dinner, or before bed.)
- **Potassium Citrate**
- **HMB** (Best taken with dinner.)
- **Glucosomine Sulfate** Great for joint pain when dealing with a Catabolic Imbalance. (Best taken with dinner.)
- **Apple Cider Vinegar** A tablespoon with meals can aid digestion. Even adding some apple cider vinegar to water that you drink throughout the day can be beneficial to a catabolic. Be cautious using apple cider vinegar as it can create loose stool issues if your bile is not flowing properly.

Avoid With This Imbalance

- **Fatty Acids like Fish or Flax Seed Oils**
- **L-Tyrosine** An amino acid.
- **Magnesium** (Including Magnesium Malate)
- **L-Taurine** An amino acid.
- **Vitamin B12**

Imbalance - Carb Burner

Often Used With This Imbalance

- **Vitamin B12** Avoid with a Catabolic Imbalance. Can help move fat into the mitochondria to be burned for fuel. (Best taken with breakfast and/or lunch. Avoid at night.)
- **Vitamin B5** Also great for breakouts if the person is not processing fats correctly - Limit use with an Anabolic Imbalance. (Best taken at night.)
- **L-Glutamine** An amino acid - Avoid with Anabolic or Electrolyte Excess Imbalances.

Avoid With This Imbalance

- **Vitamin D3**
- **L-Histadine** An amino acid.
- **Vitamin E**

Imbalance - Fat Burner

Often Used With This Imbalance

- **Magnesium Malate** Avoid with a Catabolic Imbalance. (Best taken with breakfast. Avoid at night.)
- **Vitamin A** Limit with a Catabolic Imbalance.
- **L-Taurine** An amino acid - Avoid with Electrolyte Deficiency or Catabolic Imbalances.
- **Folic Acid** Limit with an Anabolic Imbalance.
- **L-Tyrosine** An amino acid - Avoid with a Catabolic Imbalance. (Avoid at night.)

Avoid With This Imbalance

- **Vitamin B5**

Finding A Qualified Health Coach In Your Area

If you would like to find a qualified health coach who can help you with some of these supplement choices, go to www.OurCoalition.org and fill out the "Find a Health Coach" form. The Coalition will locate a health coach in your area who will contact you directly.

Wha'd He Say?

In this chapter, you learned:

- Supplements are only beneficial if you use quality products that can be assimilated by the body. Supplements improve one's health only if the supplement is appropriate for that person and his or her individual chemistry.
- Don't forget to handle digestive needs when choosing supplements.
- Once you begin using supplements, be sure to monitor your self-test numbers. When chemistry becomes more balanced, adjust the supplement protocol you are using.
- If you need supplements more intensely geared to specific imbalances, find a professional health coach in your area who has access to high-quality supplements designed to improve the imbalances discussed here.

Chapter Seventeen

Oh Yeah, Working Out

There's a reason that I waited until chapter seventeen to cover working out. I wanted to make the point loud and clear that there are sixteen other chapters that are more important. When it comes to losing weight, it's not about the workout. Working out is part of it, but time after time I see people who believe it's the whole enchilada. The reality is, it's more about the enchilada (as in... stop cramming them in your face and thinking that a good workout is going to make up for the damage you just did).

Don't forget that this is coming from a guy who makes his living by helping people work out in the gym. If this is how I make my living, yet I'm telling you this is not where your results will come from, you might want to pay attention to that piece of information. That doesn't mean that working out is worthless. Don't be silly. What I'm saying is, when it comes to results, nutrition is 90% of the pie (and it's even more effective if you leave out pie).

Do I want you to work out? Yes. I would like that very much, please. Your skinny jeans will get worn much sooner if you workout on a regular basis. What I don't want is for you to workout like you're an Olympian and neglect your diet or your imbalances altogether. You will not see the changes you envision if you skip the nutrition. As long as you understand what I'm saying, and I don't need to shake you in my kitchen again, I will share secrets to help you get the most out of your workout efforts. After all, when it comes to working out, I belong to the work smart camp and we laugh and point at the work hard camp.

I'm not going to give you a workout routine and tell you about exercises that will target your butt or abs. That's not the information that will help you the most. When it comes to types of exercises or types of workouts, those factors matter very little. What matters is the level at which you work and when and what you eat in relation to your workouts.

Nutrition According To Your Workout

First the basics:
Prior to a resistance workout, it's a good idea to eat at least something.
For an easy-to-moderate cardio workout, it's beneficial to perform this workout on an empty stomach.

Pre-Workout Nutrition For Resistance Training

For any type of anaerobic exercise, like weight lifting or high intensity movements, most people will burn glucose or glycogen. Glycogen is fuel that has been stored in the tissues and in the liver. Most people cannot burn fat for fuel while performing any of these anaerobic movements. Therefore, it's a good idea to eat something prior to a resistance workout. If you run out of glycogen, yet you continue working out, you may break down muscle tissue to use as fuel for that workout. Kind of eliminates the point of the workout, right?

Pre-Workout Nutrition For Cardio Training

Remember, some people have a harder time burning fat for fuel than others. But generally speaking, most people can burn body fat for fuel during easy-to-moderate aerobic exercise, like walking or moving in a manner that is not too strenuous. If the cardio becomes too intense, it can translate more into an anaerobic activity due to the muscular strain being placed on the body. The body can also view this vigorous activity as if you are running from a lion or some other threat. Similar to how the body reacts under stress, as the body creates glucose to use as fuel in this urgent situation, insulin levels can rise and take you out of the fat-burning mode.

A good rule to follow while attempting a fat-burning workout is this: If you are breathing too hard to carry on a normal conversation, you're working too hard to burn fat. I'm speaking generally here, but it is a nice little trick to check where you are without hooking yourself up to NASA-type body monitoring equipment while you walk around the neighborhood.

The problem is, for most individuals, if there is glucose or glycogen available, the body will always choose this fuel source over stored fat. This is why it is best to do your easy-to-moderate cardio workouts on an empty stomach. If your body can quickly burn off any glucose and/or stored glycogen at the beginning of your cardio session, it can easily move into fat-burning mode. Many believe that it takes about twenty-five minutes to burn off all your stored glycogen if you are walking or jogging moderately. If you just ate, you may first need to burn off any glucose from that food before you can dip into those glycogen stores.

The Secret Trick

In the gym, the biggest mistake I see people make is that they walk into the gym and head straight to the treadmill where they run for thirty minutes. Next, they move over to the weights and do their resistance training. They then ask me, "Why did you just smack me in the back of my head?" I go on to explain that they just burned all of their glucose and glycogen on the treadmill. They needed that fuel to perform their resistance training. With no fuel left, the body will likely break down muscle and use that for fuel since the body can't use stored fat for fuel during resistance exercises. The point of their running was to burn fat—of which they burned none —since they only burned glycogen the entire run. At this point, they usually thank me for smacking them in the back of the head.

If you just flip the order, your workout will be much more effective. This is how you work smart instead of working hard. You can warm up on the treadmill for five minutes, that's great. However, then do your resistance training while you still have glycogen stores you can use for fuel. By the time you finish your weight training (45-55 minutes later), glycogen stores will likely be depleted. Now you can hop on the treadmill and your body will be primed for burning fat. I recommend keeping your post weight training cardio to only easy walking (allowing your body to burn only fat), and limit this to a maximum of twenty-five minutes. I explain why below. You can still do hard or intense cardio on its own on a different day. Slow, easy cardio, however, is much more beneficial for weight loss after a resistance workout.

Post-Workout Nutrition For Resistance Training

After beating on your muscles, it's time to give them fuel that can be used for rebuilding. I like to use some type of protein that is easy to assimilate. A protein shake can be perfect. Please make sure you're not using anything that contains artificial sweeteners. Stevia and xylitol are okay. I prefer just stevia, but I'm okay with xylitol if that is your only option. Jay Robb and MRM brands make egg-based protein powders that I like.

However, any type of protein food source is okay too (with soft-cooked eggs being the best since a runny yolk is pro-anabolic and can aid in rebuilding muscle). I normally like to try to eat or have a shake within an hour of a resistance workout. That is why I limit any post workout cardio to only twenty-five minutes.

Post-Workout Nutrition For Cardio Training

I view my post workout nutrition for cardio the same as resistance workouts. I do, however, have one little trick. Let's say I want to do an intense cardio workout, like a spin class. I can't burn fat during that class because it is too intense. My body, however, can burn fat at a fast pace for about an hour after that class, even if I just sit on the floor and cuss about how hard that class was. With this in mind, I'll eat something about an hour before the class so I have fuel to complete the class; then I'll wait an hour or so after the class before I eat again. If I wait too long, I know my body will start breaking itself down to access fuel, so I try to eat within an hour and a half after that workout. If I immediately refuel with some type of sugary sports drink, my body will begin to burn the sugar from that drink and will not burn fat for the hour after the class.

Timing Is Everything

Timing is everything. Yet, it is also very important to simply get up off your ass and do something. Don't skip a workout because all the stars are not perfectly aligned. You can still get results eating at the wrong time, etc. I'm explaining optimal circumstances when it comes to fueling your body before and after a workout. Even though life can get in the way, don't let that get in the way of your workout. Not every workout needs to be a scientific work of art.

Start Anywhere

While trying to keep up with the salesman as you tour your local gym, the complicated equipment mocks you as you walk by. "What the heck am I supposed to do with that?" you think to yourself. "I think I saw that one at my gynecologist's office." You don't want to be that girl who climbs up onto the water fountain because she thinks it's a piece of equipment. So what do you do? You do nothing. You walk around the gym for about ten minutes hoping that at least one of the machines will resemble something from your elementary school playground so you'll know what to do with it. You eventually find yourself on a stationary bike; you get bored fifteen minutes later and head to the locker room. You go home that night, never to return, only to have $49 deducted from your checking account for the next twelve years.

I get it. The gym is intimidating and that's okay. If you don't have a friend who can show you the ropes, and you can't afford a personal trainer, start with something less flashy. Ordering a workout video online can be a great first step. Try doing a push up on your knees twice a week until you can do ten. Do a few crunches or go for a walk. Just do something. Put yourself in motion and let the possibilities create a momentum that will push you forward. In no time, you'll be at the gym, walking up to someone else on the equipment to say, "Um... your face doesn't' go there."

Resistance Training

Rest And Repair

With any type of resistance training, the benefit doesn't occur during the actual training. During the training, you're literally breaking down the body. The benefits of that workout don't show up until your body has time to repair and rebuild those muscle tissues. That is where your results come from. I have a lot of my clients see better results by reducing the number of days in a week that they work out. Personally, I give my body at least two days off per week and require my clients to take off at least one day.

Don't Repeat Muscle Groups

If you lift weights with the same muscle groups two days in a row, you just negated your efforts from the first day. For example, if you work your chest on Tuesday, the benefit from that workout would come on Wednesday when your body was repairing and rebuilding the tissues in your chest. However, if you work your chest again on Wednesday, those muscles never get the chance to rebuild and Tuesday's efforts are lost.

With resistance training, if you want to work out two days in a row, try focusing on one or two muscle groups per day. The following day, those muscles can repair while you're working other muscle groups. Here's one scenario: On Monday you work your legs, shoulders and abs. On Tuesday, you work your back and biceps. (Note: Abs and calves are the only muscle groups that some believe are okay to work two days in a row because of how those muscle fibers are structured. I still like to see a day of rest for any muscle you worked the day before. I normally work each muscle group only one time each week.) If you work your legs on Monday, it is still okay to do cardio the next day since that is not a resistance-type exercise.

Find Some Intensity

Your first workout is not the time to shoot for any type of intensity. You want to be smart and build up to any intense workout. If you injure yourself, the lack of working out while you heal could delay results. Still, as your stamina increases, you need to give your body a reason to improve.

"Pushing your body beyond its comfort zone is the trigger that creates upgrades in your physique and in your health."
                        - I just made that up

Picture doing an exercise that is very difficult for you to complete. Maybe you are doing biceps curls with a weight that is too heavy for you to complete ten reps. At that moment, your body is saying, "Okay, we can't do what this guy is trying to get us to do. We need to increase muscle fibers in his biceps so we can accomplish this task." And your body can respond by adding more muscle. If you consistently lift weights that are easy for you, your body has no reason to step it up a notch.

You still need to use good form and avoid jerking around weights that are way too heavy for you. Take the time to watch videos or learn from a professional so you understand how to use good form in your workouts. Bad form or weights that are too heavy will often result in injury.

Mixing quick and intense cardio exercises into your resistance training can also be a great way to raise intensity. Between resistance exercises, throw in a little rope jumping or sprinting on the treadmill for a minute. This is a great way to add variety to your workout. Try to keep these quick bursts to only a minute or so at a time.

Lifting Heavy Weights

A common misconception among women is that they often fear lifting weights because they don't want to look like a man. Most women do not have the chemical makeup to look like Arnold Schwarzenegger, pre-governor duties. When you see a woman who looks like Joe Piscopo just before he snapped, that woman has likely used chemical enhancements to achieve that. You're not going to lift heavy weights and have your biceps exceed the size of the Pomeranian hanging out of your purse (IT'S SO FLUFFY!). The female body is not designed to build muscle of that size, yet lifting weights heavier than those found on the sissy rack can greatly speed up weight loss. (By the way, did anyone get the fluffy reference? Anyone? Am I the only childless person who watches animated movies?)

If you are a woman who adds muscle easily or maybe your thighs get bigger and more muscular than you'd like, look at your chemistry. If you have an Anabolic Imbalance, you may be stuck in the muscle-building mode most of the time. Correcting this imbalance might allow your body to move into the breaking-down mode on a daily basis and your body won't build as much muscle.

If you're looking to add more muscle, you can also use this knowledge to watch your chemistry and implement pro-anabolic food and supplement choices to turbo charge your efforts. However, monitor your chemistry to make sure you're not pushing yourself too anabolic. You don't want to create an imbalance while you attempt to add muscle.

Interval Training

Interval training is popular and can be effective for burning fat. Intervals consist of short bursts of intense activity, followed by longer periods of very easy activity. Moving immediately back into easy activity allows the body to access stored fat for fuel, in many cases. The goal here is to burn fat during the easy activity.

Simply walk slowly for two to three minutes, then run as fast as you can for one minute. Alternate back and forth between these paces for 25-45 minutes.

Sprints

Once you've graduated from long walks and you're experimenting with some jogging, sprints can be very effective and take the least amount of time. I'm not going to get into a lot of the science here, but many believe that short sprints are a much better choice for your body than long runs. When I do sprints, I try to do four sprints, each for one minute, running as fast as I can. I rest for a few minutes between each sprint. This can allow you to perform an effective cardio session in about twelve minutes. That's the whole workout. Be sure you are warmed up and stretched before you sprint. The goal here is to strengthen your heart, increase your body's metabolism and reduce the amount of fat your body stores throughout the day. Like I said, the science behind this one is a whole other book. In any case, it is still very simple to execute.

Don't Starve Yourself After A Workout

If your body is repairing and rebuilding muscle tissue the day following your workout, what do you think happens if you skip breakfast? If you're not bringing in the nutrients needed to build tissue, not only are you missing out on increasing muscle fibers, you're likely going to lose muscle. When the body needs more resources, it will break down muscle tissues (among other necessary parts) to get what it needs. How effective does that make the previous day's workout? Not so much. Unless Oprah was playing on the gym TV and you used that time to soak in her beauty (I think if you mention in your book how pretty Oprah is, she invites you to be a guest on her show... Dr. Oz, you're pretty too).

"When you work your body, give your body what it needs to rebuild your body."
- Guy who overuses the word "body"

Imbalances And Working Out

A strong imbalance can also affect the level at which you should be working out.

<u>Electrolyte Deficiency Imbalance</u>

With an Electrolyte Deficiency Imbalance, your resources are likely already low. View your nutrient and mineral reserves as money in the bank and every workout is costing you money. It's still okay to work out, in most cases. Simply be aware that working out too much could leave you depleted and allow The Psycho Factor to show up. However, if you limit your workouts to what your body can handle, and make an attempt to further increase minerals and nutrients on the days you workout, you can successfully incorporate exercise into your life. Increasing medium-carb foods on your workout day is a good idea in these cases.

<u>Catabolic Imbalance</u>

Any form of working out is pro-catabolic, at least a little bit. If a strong Catabolic Imbalance showed on your *Imbalance Guide*, working out too often might cause you to exacerbate that imbalance and fall apart. The right thing to do when dealing with a strong Catabolic Imbalance is to reduce your workout load or increase your pro-anabolic food choices or supplement protocol.

People with a Catabolic Imbalance should also try to work out in the morning, or at least before 3PM when possible. With this plan, they will at least be pushing themselves more catabolic during the day, when they are intended to be catabolic.

If you have an Anabolic Imbalance, increasing your number of workouts per week may help you correct that imbalance. I still like to see a person take at least one entire day off per week. However, due to your body being stuck in the rebuilding mode, the breakdown that comes with working out won't be as detrimental to you as it can be to someone dealing with a Catabolic Imbalance.

Sweating

Yes. Do some sweating. There is a reason your body sweats. While working out, there is an increase in lactic acid production and all sorts of other craziness going on. We sweat so the body has a way to remove these acids so they don't accumulate and create havoc. When you work out in front of a fan, or cold air conditioner, you're restricting your body's ability to sweat out this junk. Don't do that.

Sweating is another strategy your body uses to remove junk. By allowing your body to sweat, you can speed up weight loss by reducing the load of acids and other chemical reactions that the body has to deal with. There is a point where a person can overheat. That's not what I want you to do. However, allowing your body to sweat during a workout can have many benefits.

If you're someone who never sweats, your pores may be clogged up and that could be contributing to your weight gain. Go to a dry or steam sauna to see if you can pop the corks, so to speak, in those pores and allow you to start sweating. If you have an Electrolyte Deficiency Imbalance, keep in mind that the body sweats out minerals while it is sweating out junk. Therefore, don't spend too much time in any type of sauna until you raise your mineral levels.

Wha'd He Say?

In this chapter, you learned:

- For most people, working out will equate to only 10% of your results. 90% of your results will likely come from what you eat and how your body processes those foods.
- Prior to a resistance workout, it's a good idea to eat something.

- For an easy-to-moderate, fat-burning, cardio workout, it's beneficial to perform this workout on an empty stomach.
- After warming up, start your workout with resistance training and do any easy cardio afterwards.
- Women should not be afraid of lifting heavy weights. The muscles created will help you burn fat faster and create that lean look.
- Starving yourself after a workout can eliminate the benefits of that workout.

CHAPTER EIGHTEEN

A Healthy Body In An Unhealthy World

Nobody can avoid everything that is bad for the human body. It's just not possible in the world we live in. Even if you cancel your DirecTV subscription, fire your dog walker, and move out into the woods, you can still have a bird fly over and poop in your mouth while you're sunbathing next to a natural stream. The trick is not to try to eliminate every toxin, chemical and pollutant from entering your body; but, instead, to put your body in a position where it can have an easier time of removing those problems. That's the whole point in improving the "flow" of the body and balancing the systems that make it all work.

While you're helping your body perform at a higher level, the next goal is to merely learn about the facets of your life that are contributing to your body's toxic load, then get rid of the ones that are the easiest for you to eliminate. Don't feel like you need to run in horror from every environmental or household pollutant within a thirty-mile radius or you're going to be doing some Forrest Gump-type running. However, if there are factors in your life that are easy for you to change, go ahead and change them. That will be one less irritant that your body has to deal with—one less task that it needs to take care of before it can move on to more important bodily processes.

It's my view that the body was designed to handle some of this junk. Worrying about every possible toxin is just going to create more stress, more harmful chemicals that accompany that stress, and more work for your body to do. Criminy Pete! Chill out and enjoy your life.

In this chapter, I also talk about items that many people feel are healthy solutions and why they may be misguided. Bear in mind that almost every product, method or idea out there could benefit *somebody*. I think there are very few ideas that are completely invalid for the entire population. I just get annoyed when people try to push their products on everyone and market their products as if they are the solution to every human ailment existing today. I feel strongly that there is no such product; a lot of it has to do with what happens to be popular at any given moment. I mean, now it seems popular to watch shows about people getting screamed at in a kitchen. Who saw that coming?

Before I dive into this chapter, I'd like to pause and reflect on a few things:

1. Don't treat your symptoms and don't use symptoms to label yourself with an imbalance.
2. Get help. This work can get very complicated. If you run into trouble, find a health coach in your area who can help you.
3. I just want to point out that I've completed more than seventeen chapters of this book without once making fun of Paris Hilton or Snookie. Sometimes, I amaze even myself.

Chemicals In Tap Water

I was at my brother's house in Florida this summer when we decided to use his pool testing kit to look at his tap water. We tested both his pool and the water from the tap in his kitchen. We both sort of freaked when we saw that there was more chlorine in his tap water than in his pool! What the...?! My brother freaked because he thought, "Man, I must really need more chlorine in my pool," and ran out to his shed to add more. But his pool wasn't green with algae; and it became clear the next day, as all of our eyes were burning in the pool during a game of paddle ball, that he really didn't need more chlorine in his pool—he needed less in his tap water.

Most city water treatment plants use both chlorine and fluoride to treat the water. Both of these chemicals are harmful to the human body in their own right. An immediate impact these chemicals can have on the body is their ability to "displace" iodine from the body. I say "displace" because that is how most researchers view what chlorine and fluoride are doing to iodine levels in the body. Though iodine levels do normally go down if consuming chlorine- and fluoride-laden water, I view this another way: Iodine acts as a disperser in the body. It disperses toxins so they can be removed from the system. The body views chlorine and fluoride as toxins. (Yes, I know your dentist told you fluoride was good for your teeth, but what he didn't tell you is that it is not good for your body... oops. He will also tell you mercury in your mouth isn't dangerous.) Therefore, iodine is used to help disperse these toxins. In essence, these chemicals are stripping, or displacing, the iodine from the system, but it makes more sense to view this as the body is just using up its iodine to deal with this problem. In any event, an iodine deficiency can be created.

It is widely accepted that iodine is required for proper thyroid function, and thyroid "conditions" have been on the rise in the past decade or so. Although I feel that the rise of this epidemic has more to do with the rise in popularity of prescribing thyroid medications, it could also be partially due to the fact that cities are using more and more chemicals to treat our water. It is also important to consider that iodine is a mineral that can be difficult for some people to absorb. Some minerals are easier to absorb than others and come into the system even if the system is imbalanced. Iodine, on the other hand, requires a more balanced pH in the system in order to be absorbed properly. That's why giving iodine to patients with thyroid issues will often bring no result. You can dump all the iodine you want into a person; but if that iodine can't be absorbed, it's not going to help. This is why the medical world has shifted to using drugs in most thyroid cases.

The significance of this, in reference to water, is understanding that if people already have a low level of iodine, you can see how drinking tap water filled with chlorine or fluoride could really do a number on their iodine levels. Crazy to see how just drinking tap water could result in a thyroid issue, right? Yet, understanding the science makes it hard to argue.

Most filter pitchers filter the water through carbon which does very little to remove these chemicals from your tap water. When it comes to filters, I like the good reverse osmosis filters that can be installed under your sink; but even these filters can remove good minerals while they're removing the bad stuff. If you use a reverse osmosis filter, it's a good idea to add mineral drops back into your water. The company, Trace Minerals Research, makes a product called Concentrace Trace Mineral Drops. It's sold at most health food stores. Adding just three or four drops per glass of water can replenish minerals that may have been stripped during the filtration process. Of course, if you have high blood pressure, you would cut that dosage in half.

Spring water is the best option, but it can be costly to buy. I don't really like the idea of distilled water for most people because it is void of any mineral whatsoever, and can wash away more mineral than spring water might. For some people, merely getting any form of water into them is going to be beneficial; so again, I don't want to split hairs with water for some. But since I'm talking about ways to reduce the intake of toxic substances, the type of water can be important.

Shower Filters

Now that you understand the trouble that chlorine can cause, let's hit the showers because most of us don't think about how the water we bathe in can affect our bodies. It's true that most of us don't drink the water coming out of the showerhead while we're washing our hair, but we do continue to breathe while we're showering. When that hot water turns into mist and steam, it still contains all the chemicals that are in that water. As we breathe in this steam, those chemicals come into our lungs then into our bloodstream even faster than if we were drinking the water. In a way, this could make the need to filter our shower water even more important than filtering the water we're drinking. Since this water has a faster path to your bloodstream, doing something to remove or reduce this chlorine can be a good idea.

This is a pretty easy fix and I have had a lot of people tell me how much better they started feeling after they added a shower filter. I myself was getting extremely tired after my showers and the only thought I could come up with was, "How long was I in there?!" I never considered that the steam in my shower was filling my lungs with chemicals that my body was scrambling to figure out how to remove. You can buy a shower filter for about $40 at most health food stores. You just screw it onto the shower's water source between the pipe coming out of the wall and the shower head itself and you're done. You can even buy replacement filters for less so you don't have to buy a new filter system every time.

These shower filters usually run the water through carbon. We already know how that won't remove enough chlorine and fluoride to make water suitable for drinking. In this regard, we know these shower filters are not likely removing all the chemicals from the water. But with such an easy and inexpensive step, you can at least begin to reduce the amount of chemicals in your showering experience. For a lot of people, this simple step can reduce the load on their bodies and bring some relief. I hope I didn't scare you away from showering and your plan is to simply stink from now on.

Microwaves

Much of this book has been about correcting issues to allow your body to use the food you're eating and improve its ability to remove junk and synthetic substances that your body can't process. That's why microwaves are an important topic. If you're going to correct your digestion so that you can actually pull the nutrients out of the food you eat, the food you eat should be something that your body can use. Too many sources have scared me away from using microwaves. It is believed that the way microwaves heat food is a process that changes the molecular structure of the food in order to create the friction that makes it hot. When you change the molecular structure of a natural food, it can become unrecognizable to the body and the body may not be able to process it correctly.

There are as many studies that show this to be false as there are studies that show this problem to be true. Is it easier to heat something in the microwave? Of course it is. But you need to understand: If anything heated by a microwave not only loses its nutritional value to the body, but also becomes a problem that the body has to deal with, that is not worth the risk to me. It will take you longer to prepare your food without a microwave; but it could be time that you save in the long run by reducing the number of doctor and hospital visits you need to make. I just use my microwave as a very fancy clock.

You may still be skeptical and thinking, "Okay Tony, I'll fix my digestion, but why ya gotta mess with my Hot Pockets?" I'll give you a little experiment. Go down to Home Depot and buy two identical potted plants. Name one plant "Ricky" and the other one "Reject Plant-Child." I guess you can pick your own names if you want. In any case, take them home and put them in the same light. Water one plant with normal water, and the other plant with water that has been microwaved. Don't pour the hot water in the plant because obviously that won't go well. Just microwave some water and let it cool to room temperature before you water with it.

At the end of your experiment, I think you will find that one plant is happy, while the other plant has earned the name I suggested. Many believe that microwaves can even change the structure of water and turn it into an evil substance.

Many chain restaurants have switched over to cooking all of their food in microwaves. Food is shipped in bags and the "cooks" simply pop the bags in the microwave. The only cooking they do is in the deep fryer. Are ya kiddin' me? If I was in the boardroom when they made that decision, you would have heard a world of cussing.

What Am I Cooking In?

To keep this brief, understand that what you cook with counts. If you're cooking in plastics, aluminum, or typical "non-stick" cookware, some of these poisons are off-gassing into your food and into your body. This creates another toxin that your body has to deal with. Some of these heavy metal toxins don't have an exit strategy from the body and can accumulate and cause all types of trouble. Glass is always safe to cook with or drink out of, stainless steel is rarely suspect. Enamel cookware is also considered to be safer than most non-stick cookware.

What's In My Mouth?

The medical field is not the only world that practically gives us a "daily allowance" of toxins. We learned in the middle of the 18th century that mercury is poison and nothing has changed since—mercury is still poison. After the dentist finishes putting mercury into someone's teeth, he takes what is left over and puts it in a special container marked "hazardous materials." That container then goes into another container marked "hazardous materials." Next, a little truck that has the special markings and permits required to haul hazardous materials comes and picks up that mercury from the dentist's office. And of course the ADA doctors will still tell you it's safe to put mercury in your mouth and let it seep into your head 24 hours a day. Dental work that is toxic, medications that are toxic—with all this disclosure I feel like I'm breaking the news to Honey Boo Boo that there is no Easter Bunny.

Smoking

Smoking? Seriously? I don't really need to explain this, do I? I think you understand that you'll need to stop smoking to have any chance of improving your health. People think that smoking just affects the lungs, but it also puts a lot of tar and chemicals in the body that need to be filtered out by the liver. As I said in an earlier chapter, the two most important factors in health, in my opinion, are digestion and liver function. We aren't what we eat—we are what we can assimilate and what we can't remove. If your liver is overwhelmed, the body is having a hard time removing all the junk that should be removed. If it can't be removed, the junk will be stored in joints, tissues, or fat cells.

Here's the good news: The people who have a difficult time trying to quit smoking are almost always people with a low mineral content. The nicotine and the chemicals thicken blood and constrict the vascular system to raise blood pressure. So, when people with no mineral identity try to quit, it can sometimes be hard for them because smoking was helping to lift their blood pressure. If you are a smoker and your *Imbalance Guide* shows that you may be dealing with an Electrolyte Deficiency Imbalance, losing the smokes might just be a whole lot easier when you improve this imbalance. You're still going to have to want to quit. It's not going to be magic, but it will make it physiologically easier. Understanding how the body works can change the viewpoint of choices that we make in our lives. This new understanding can reveal that a bad habit could actually be a form of self-medication. The exciting part is that the bad habit is easier to get rid of when it no longer represents the main choice for the "medication." To learn more, you will soon be able to check out *Done With Smoking*.

Antibiotics

Antibiotics don't just break apart the bad bacteria in your body; they also break apart all the good bacteria that live in your intestines. These good bacteria do these good things: Help with digestion, control infestation from yeast and bad bacteria like candida, make the B vitamins we need, and help clean putrefied fecal matter off of colon walls. When we take antibiotics and wipe out all the good bacteria along with the bad, we need to replace the good bacteria with probiotics. Yet our doctors don't normally teach us how to do this.

215

Here's another issue many people, like me, have with antibiotics: Many antibiotics are actually made from fungus. When you use these antibiotics to kill a bacterial or viral problem, you're actually setting up the terrain of the body in a way that allows fungal problems to flourish. Imagine you have a garden and weeds are taking over in a big way. Would you try to eliminate those weeds by planting new weeds that were designed to kill the original weeds? That sentence alone sounds horribly dumb just from the number of times "weeds" showed up. If the sentence sounds stupid, obviously the idea is not that brilliant. If you want to get rid of a problem, it might be a good idea to use a method that isn't going to end up creating another problem.

Flu Shots

Ignorant.

Alkalizing Water And Water Filters

In the marketplace today, there is a lot of information about "alkalizing" that is a heaping pile of fiction. I don't cover the Acid and Alkaline Imbalances in this book, but I do include them in Appendix C. However, if you are currently using, or plan to use any alkalizing products or alkalizing water, be sure to read about them in Appendix C. It's very important that you understand if these products are right for you or not.

Wha'd He Say?

In this chapter, you learned:

- The trick is not to try to eliminate every toxin, chemical and pollutant from entering your body. Instead, work to put your body in a position where it can have an easier time removing those toxins.
- Use your microwave as a clock, and nothing else.
- You're not still smoking, are you?

CHAPTER NINETEEN

Will The Diets Ever Stop?!

Why Popular Diets Don't Work For Everyone

This is my favorite part of the whole book (outside of that time when I was really funny). I love it when people learn enough science to understand why the diets they tried before didn't work for them. They usually cuss a little bit, thinking back to all the time they wasted counting calories, or juicing a turkey sandwich, or scouring the countryside looking for some hoggelwart herb that was going to make the fat fall off. It's okay to be annoyed about the bad advice you got, but the real lesson here is that your failures probably make sense—and they were probably not your fault. Even better, now you're going to understand what to do to either make that diet work for you or put together a plan that is right for your body and your biological makeup.

Here I break down popular diets and explain why they work for some people and not for others. In each section I group a few diets together. I understand there are variations between the diets I am grouping together, but the major malfunction is the same—so this will save time.

My explanations do not mean that these are all bad diets. You get that by now, right? It just means that they are not right for everyone, as the creators of these diets often indicate.

I may repeat a few nuggets I have already explained in this book because I want to freak you out when you realize how much you understand now.

Low-Fat Diets

<u>When Do These Diets Work?</u>

The low-fat diet craze hit in the eighties and we're still paying the price today. The fact that we were all walking around in parachute pants carrying giant boom boxes on our shoulders should have clued us in to the fact that we didn't know what the heck we were doing. Alas, Members Only jackets were everywhere, Molly Ringwald still rose to fame and so did the low-fat diet.

You've had a hard time getting me to shut up about bile flow in this book; but if people have reduced or restricted bile flow, they have a hard time emulsifying and processing dietary fats. If those fats can't be processed correctly, they can turn toxic in the body. These toxic fats can be pushed out of the body through the skin, creating horrible acne issues; or the body can store these undigested fats in fat cells, and these people become round.

By removing fats from the diet, these individuals with poor bile flow can remove a burden from the body. Now, those fats don't have to be stored in fat cells and these people can lose weight.

<u>When Do These Diets Fail?</u>

When fats are reduced, something else must be increased. We calculate food by looking at fats, carbs and proteins. If we reduce fats, carbs or proteins must increase. You already learned how higher levels of carbs can spike insulin levels and signal the body to store fat. You also learned that the body needs appropriate fats to perform specific functions in the body. If your diet doesn't include fats that are appropriate for you, your body will be less likely to let go of stored fat.

This is my least favorite diet for many reasons that I've already discussed in this book. Most diet books written in the past ten years agree with me so I won't beat this one into the ground anymore.

Low-Calorie Diets

When Do These Diets Work?

These diets work when you have horrible goals. If your goal is to lose weight on the scale, yet you have no concern for long-term weight gain or long-term health in any way, this is the diet for you (keep in mind that I'm talking like an idiot and at no point will these diets ever be good). When you starve yourself with a low-calorie diet, you're not losing only body fat. In most cases, you're losing muscle as well. In this regard, the scale may tell you that you've lost weight, yet you still feel as mushy as you did before the diet. The loss of muscle will also slow your metabolism and set you up for drastic weight gain the minute you snap and decide you can't live your life eating only four bowls of cabbage soup each day.

The main reason a low-calorie diet can be successful is because it makes you conscious of what you're eating. If you need to track everything you eat in order to gauge if you stayed within your calorie limit, this forces you to look at what you eat each day. It's amazing to see people start journaling their food only to realize, "Wow, I never noticed I drink eleven sodas each day." Also, a lot of processed junk food has higher calories than real food. So, to stay within the limits, dieters will start eating more real food. This will almost always lead to weight loss.

A low-calorie diet can create weight loss only if a person can access stored fat and burn it for fuel. However, remember that it can be difficult for some people to burn stored fat for fuel because their bodies are predisposed to burn glucose. This is normally dependent on the type of calories being consumed, not the number of calories. Most low-calorie diets simply have you count the calories. There is a big difference between 800 calories of chicken and spinach and 800 calories of chocolate chip cookies.

Wow, I really didn't have many positive things to say about these diets in the *When Do These Diets Work?* section. I hate to see what happens when I begin to explain the bad sides of the low-calorie diets.

When Do These Diets Fail?

Almost always. Many people can lose weight initially, but the weight often returns. When you starve the body and fail to provide the nutrients that it needs, the body will steal those nutrients from tissues and bones. If you want to freak out a woman today, just mention osteoporosis. Osteoporosis should not be considered a disease in which the body "attacks" its own bones. The body is breaking down bone to access needed minerals that are not coming into the system. This is most commonly due to digestive issues, yet starving yourself can create the same result.

You can not only break down muscles, tissues, or bones while you're on a low calorie diet, you may break down organ tissues as well. It is very common for the body to pull protein out of our lungs when enough protein is not coming into the system. Here's a hint: You need your lungs.

Starving yourself will only set you up for immediate and drastic weight gain the moment you start to eat regularly. It's not a fun game.

Low-Carb Diets

<u>When Do These Diets Work?</u>

Low-carb diets allow people to keep insulin levels low, giving their bodies an opportunity to burn stored fat for fuel. That is the idea I've been pushing through this whole book. However, not all low-carb diets are created equal. Before I examine the differences, let's first look at when low-carb diets don't work.

<u>When Do These Diets Fail?</u>

If you reduce carbs, you need to increase fats and/or proteins. If you have digestive issues, this will be a problem. If you have poor bile flow and can't process fats correctly, the increase in fat intake could lead to weight gain. If you can't fully break down proteins, rotting and fermented foods are going to lead to weight gain. So, even if you're keeping your insulin levels low, but unprocessed fats or proteins are junking up the system, you could have a hard time losing weight. You may even gain weight.

Don't forget The Psycho Factor. If people using a low-carb diet have low mineral levels and low blood pressure, they need to include carbs or sugars to buffer those low mineral levels. These people would first need to lift their mineral levels or correct any digestive issues before they could use a low-carb diet without becoming miserable.

Variations In Low-Carb Diets

Processed junk food can be a big factor in low-carb diets. Many of these diets promote the use of low-carb snack foods and processed meals. Many contain artificial sweeteners that are toxic to the body (and we know that means those toxins can be stored as fat). I always prefer to see people eat real food over a processed food, even if it is low-carb.

Eating Paleo

The Paleo Diet is currently the fastest growing diet in popularity. There are variations within the paleo world; but, generally speaking, if a caveman ate it, you can eat it on a paleo diet. Do me a favor and avoid picturing your plate with a big hunk of meat and a handful of twigs. That's not what a Paleo Diet is all about. It's about eating real food and avoiding processed foods like grains, dairy and things you might find in a vending machine.

When it comes to what I personally eat, a Paleo Diet is closer than anything else out there. However, I eat that way because it's the right choice for me, not because it's the right choice for everyone. I also add variations that are beneficial to my chemistry. I tend to lean more catabolic so I consume a lot of butter and heavy cream to help push myself more anabolic. This is okay with some paleo experts, but a big no-no with others. Again, I do what's right for my digestive strength and my body chemistry, not because I'm following a popular diet.

Though I feel a Paleo Diet is the most optimal diet plan out there, it still has the same troubles most low-carb diet plans have. I don't really view paleo as a low-carb diet, because that is not the focus; but it does turn out to be very low in carbs since grains are removed.

If a person has digestive issues and can't handle the proteins or the fats included in a Paleo Diet, this diet will also be unsuccessful for him. You still need to look at yourself and how your body is processing foods to know if you can process the foods that make up any eating plan.

Vegan, Vegetarian, and Meat-Free Diets

When Do These Diets Work?

Vegetarian-based diets are often successful because they contain a lot of green vegetables. Green, non-starch vegetables have tremendous nutritional upside. Therefore, if your diet contains a lot of vegetables, many benefits can follow, including weight loss.

In chapter thirteen I discussed how animal proteins are harder to digest than vegetables or even grains. If people have poor digestion, they will feel much better once they remove animal protein from their diet. This can be beneficial in the beginning until they run out of their reserve of nutrients that can only be found in animal sources.

When Do These Diets Fail?

These diets fail when a person believes that as long as something is vegan, it must be healthy. When people eliminate meat, they often increase carbohydrates and other processed foods. These people also often eat a lot of processed meat replacement products. Many meat replacement products are made predominantly of soy. I have already discussed how too much soy can affect estrogen levels in the body.

Once an individual has been avoiding animal products for long enough (this can be different for every person), problems can arise from the lack of nutrients that can only be found in animal products. A B12 shot is not enough to remedy these deficiencies.

Juicing Diets

When Do These Diets Work?

Juicing allows people to obtain vitamins and minerals from a variety of foods without having to digest those foods. If a person is dealing with digestive issues, juicing can bring an immediate lift and help him feel better. It can also remove the burden of having to digest food. This can aid in weight loss by freeing the body up to handle other issues, like excess toxins that need to be removed.

If an individual has strong insulin, and can process the sugars in the juice without too much of an insulin spike, weight loss can occur.

<u>When Do These Diets Fail?</u>

When you juice a food, fruit for example, you remove all the fiber. The fiber is there to decrease how quickly those sugars hit your bloodstream. Without any fiber, the sugars from the fruit hit the bloodstream quickly and spike insulin levels. If you are leaning toward insulin resistance, that can be bad news for weight loss.

If you try to incorporate resistance training with a juicing diet, you may find it difficult to add muscle. Without the protein needed to build muscle, your efforts in the gym could be wasted. Since juicing doesn't do anything to correct digestive issues, most people who do see results from a juicing diet will gain that weight back once they return to eating food.

Wha'd He Say?

In this chapter, you learned:

- There is no diet that is right for everybody.

CHAPTER TWENTY (THE SUM UP)

Review & Make Your Plan

Now What?

I want to take a moment to lay out the important points that I've covered so you have an easy reference you can use to put your plan together. I know this was a lot of information and you may feel a little overwhelmed and excited at the same time. Just take a deep breath and I'll cover the important points that you don't want to forget and a few that will help you move forward and avoid pitfalls.

You've learned an incredible amount of information so this section will be where I pull a Mr. Miyagi and help you put it all together in a usable format. By the end of this wrap-up, you should be saying, "Ah, that's why he had me painting his fence."

Bring It All Together

Achieving lasting weight loss is most commonly about the foods that you are eating and how your body is processing those foods. Correcting any digestive issues or imbalances will greatly speed up your results.

Here are major points to remember:

1. Correct any digestive issues so you can pull needed resources out of the food you're eating. DON'T SKIP THIS.
2. Ensure you are pooping it up real nice. A stool that is too hard and leaning toward constipation or too loose and leaning toward diarrhea needs to be corrected. Both constipation and diarrhea can lead to weight gain for different reasons.

3. Reduce starch and carbohydrate intake to keep insulin levels on an even keel. This will allow your body to burn stored fat as fuel.
4. Don't let cravings derail your efforts. Watch your self-test numbers and take the necessary steps if cravings are calling your name.
5. Work toward correcting any imbalances that may be causing weight gain.
6. Don't be afraid of fats in your diet. Be sure, however, that your bile is flowing well enough to process those fats. If you're not sure, use a beet and beet greens product to get your bile flowing.
7. If mineral levels and blood pressure are low, use medium-carb foods to fight off cravings while you bring up your mineral levels (either by correcting digestion or adding unrefined salt and other mineral lifting supplements).
8. Don't skip breakfast and send your body into starvation mode.

These are some of the most important steps for lasting weight loss. Since you have read this book, measured where your chemistry is, and understand how to monitor yourself, you know which of the foregoing factors apply to you the most. Since everyone is different, some of the points may not be as important or even apply to you. Remember, this book is about figuring out your specific cause for weight gain. It isn't about reading a bunch of stuff and then just following the summary list at the end. It's about responding to measurements. You can't manage what you don't measure. Pay attention to where you are and make adjustments accordingly.

Fix Digestive Issues

By reviewing your *Digestive Issue Validators* on your *Imbalance Guide*, you know if you need to put some attention toward improving digestion. Odds are great that if you're reading this book, you do. **Don't skip this step. You will not get the results you want if you don't improve digestion through supplementation.** I have seen people improve imbalances using only food and lifestyle choices; but very few will correct digestive issues without the aid of supplements, at least temporarily. If you're not digesting food successfully, and your body is not getting the resources it needs, losing weight and keeping it off will be more difficult. Digestion is huge. Don't skip it.

Correct Your Imbalances

Taking steps toward correcting an imbalance and *actually* correcting an imbalance are not the same thing. To Improve symptoms requires correcting the imbalance that is causing those symptoms. If you take steps to correct an Electrolyte Deficiency Imbalance, but your blood pressure is still incredibly low and all your numbers are still pointing to an Electrolyte Deficiency Imbalance, then more needs to be done to correct the issue.

You don't want to be the guy who says, "I did what you told me to do and I'm still overweight." Put more stock in your numbers than in what you are doing to correct them. If your self-test numbers still show an imbalance, the symptoms will often still be there to go right along with that imbalance. Just because you did some work to correct the imbalance doesn't mean that you did ENOUGH work to correct YOUR imbalance. For some, it will take more effort and more time to see the results and move the body closer to balance. If you are experiencing a stubborn imbalance, get help from a professional who can guide you. You're probably just missing a key point or doing things to work against yourself as you try to create improvements.

Monitor Your Numbers

Monitoring is a crucial step. When a person starts feeling better, it becomes easy to forget why this improvement came to be. I see a lot of clients who do the work to see improvement and then they stop doing the right things, go back to their old habits, and wonder why their issues or their weight comes back. You wouldn't workout for one month, lose a little weight and expect that weight to continue to stay off if you stopped working out. You have to continue to be aware of how your body is operating if you want to continue to see results. Yes, the amount of monitoring you'll need to do may drastically decrease once the body is in balance. Monitoring less frequently will certainly be appropriate once you're feeling great. But you still need to check your numbers from time to time and make sure everything is going as planned. This will allow you to steer clear of many problems.

Don't Work Against Yourself

Taking steps in the right direction is absolutely the most important way to get started. However, the steps you take in the wrong direction still count. Continuing to eat a lot of sugar or starches is still going to spike insulin levels for most people and cause fat to be stored.

Don't forget that you now have the tools to correct the cravings that cause you to eat all that junk. By correcting those cravings, reducing starches and sugars becomes a lot easier.

Try to remember that there is already a lot working against you, and it is likely not your fault that you are dealing with these issues. I feel like the despicable farming methods used in this country have to be responsible for a lot of our deficiencies. You may feel people shouldn't have to work this hard at living, and you're right; but profiteering in the farming industry is a reality. Keep this in the back of your mind in case your issues return, so you can become vigilant again about taking the right steps. In the same way that it can be fun to grow a nice plant, it can also be enjoyable to continue feeling better and having more vitality.

Make Your Plan

If you fail to plan, you plan to fail. Is it a little annoying that I said that? Yes, it is. But if it gets you to put together a course of action, I'm okay with being annoying. It doesn't take much for life to get in the way. The good news is that any time your pants start to feel a little tight, you can use that as a reminder that you have yet to take the time to make the needed improvements. Writing up a plan in a notebook can help you avoid that reminder.

Since what you eat counts, know what you're going to eat before it's time to eat. If you wait until you're starving to decide what you're going to eat that day, you're going to end up with a scoop of Golden Grahams in a taco shell. Once major hunger strikes, all proper judgment can go out the window. Plan what you're going to eat ahead of time and you will make better choices.

In a similar vein, grocery stores have a magic threshold that erases your brain as you walk in the sliding glass doors. Know what you're going to buy before you get there.

If you find that you need to use supplements to improve digestion or an imbalance, plan that as well. Most of us live our lives on the go. Burger King doesn't carry the supplements you need, so you can't just drive through and grab them while you're out. Success will take making some new habits, but if you plan ahead, everything gets easier.

You're not going to make just one plan and stick with that forever. Remember that your plan will be adjusted as the measurements change on your *Data Tracking Sheet*.

Avoid Self Sabotage

There really is no such thing as a "side effect"—only direct effects. When you use a supplement or change your diet, or increase or decrease water intake... all these things have the ability to change your body chemistry, and that change can create an effect. It's not a side effect; you did something and things changed. It's a direct effect.

I have heard "side effect" described as choosing to put up with poisonous or negative effects in order to have a particular benefit. Don't you think the better choice is to have only benefit? Let's choose the positive without the price of a negative.

Avoid looking at these changes like, "This doesn't work for me," and therefore quit trying to balance your body. Whatever change you are creating is just more information. If something creates the opposite reaction than what you're looking for, then you can use that information to steer in the right direction. If you understand how to look at the clues, you don't have to jump ship just because a bird pooped on the deck of the boat.

If you choose a course of action, and your measurements show things going in the opposite direction, try to remember that a change in measurement that goes in the opposite direction is still wonderful information. You're finding your way. If a supplement or food choice doesn't work, that information can go a long way in determining what WILL work for you. Why did a choice push you in the opposite direction? Use that information to look for an answer. Find a practitioner to help you decipher why anything might push you in the wrong direction. If you need help but can't afford it, join the free community described below, and post questions to see if other community members have experience with similar situations.

Here are two examples. A young man by the name of Soupy was having stomach pains. (Good thing I changed his name for this book. That would have been very unfortunate if his name was really Soupy.) Soupy's body was not creating enough stomach acid to break down the food he was eating. As his food would rot and ferment, gases were created that would expand his intestines and cause pain and bloating. He started using HCL supplements and immediately his pain began to reduce. But he also started experiencing painful heartburn.

You may not know that the LES (Lower Esophageal Sphincter) valve at the bottom of the esophagus is triggered to close when stomach acid levels rise due to digestion kicking in. Without enough stomach acid, that valve doesn't close and you can have reflux. If there is no stomach acid, you won't even feel that reflux because there is no acid coming up to burn you (you can learn more about this in Appendix A). If you begin to add HCL supplementation, now you have some acid in your stomach. But if you haven't reached a high enough dose to trigger that valve to close, now you have reflux that contains acid and you get burned. This can happen even if you are avoiding starches while you initially begin increasing HCL intake (as explained in chapter three.)

Soupy thought that since he had never experienced heartburn before, it must be the HCL that was giving him heartburn so he stopped using it. If he had just increased his dosage according to instructions, his acid levels would have triggered the valve to close, reflux would stop and he could have continued receiving the relief from his stomach pains that follow every meal for him. By misunderstanding what his body was telling him, he missed an opportunity to improve his health and eliminate a horrible discomfort he lives with every day.

Another example is what happened to Sugarplum. Yes, her name really is Sugarplum. Sugarplum wanted to correct her Electrolyte Deficiency Imbalance and also lose weight. She began using supplements to improve her imbalance and correct her digestion. She lowered her carb intake so her insulin would not spike as often and cause her body to store fat. This helped her to drop weight.

But her cravings for sugar also began to skyrocket. She had never had uncontrollable cravings before so she assumed that the supplements she was using had messed up her body in some way and caused her to be a sugar freak so she stopped taking supplements. This is a fun deduction, but as an option, we could also use science and logic to figure out what happened to Sugarplum.

You learned earlier that cravings are mostly created from low minerals and/or low blood sugar. Sugarplum was taking the right steps to improve her Electrolyte Deficiency Imbalance but her imbalance was strong and her blood pressure was still extremely low, indicating that she still had a low level of minerals in her system. Once she lowered her carb and sugar intake to lose weight, there was now nothing left to buffer the system—not enough minerals and not enough sugars. Cravings almost always skyrocket when sugars and minerals are both low.

Before she started attempting to raise her mineral levels with supplements, she never had cravings because she was buffering her system with carbs and sugars (which is the reason she had gained weight in the first place). As long as sugars are high, a person won't get those cravings. Weight gain often shows up as a result of keeping those sugars high, but the uncontrollable cravings can be kept at bay.

If Sugarplum would have added some medium-carb foods (not starch) to her diet, instead of eliminating all carbs, the sugars from those carbs could have continued to buffer her low mineral content. Her weight loss would have been more gradual, but that's okay since she would also be keeping her cravings away. As her mineral content and blood pressure began to climb, she could have reduced her carbs further at that point if she still needed to lose weight. The important lesson here is not to look at the changes you make as "not working" or "causing crazy side effects." As I said, these were all direct effects—not side effects. These effects just needed to be looked at logically so she could use them to steer her next move.

The moral of both these examples is this: Avoid Self Sabotage. Most people never have an opportunity to correct the issues that are plaguing them. Don't ruin that opportunity because you decide to ignore how your system works. Listen to the clues that show up. If they don't make sense to you, get help from someone who can help you decipher them. Stay determined and keep in mind why you started this journey. You can be *Done With Being Fat* if you're willing to just do the work. Do a self-test. Measure your numbers so your situation will make sense to you. Then, you can regulate what is needed.

Finding Supplements

Remember, a lot of the supplements I talk about in this book will not be found in stores. Most products that I talk about in this book can be found on www.NaturalReference.com. Don't forget about digestion when ordering supplements. If you're like most of the readers of this book, digestion will be the priority and you will likely be ordering Betaine HCL, Beet Flow, and Digesti-zyme to cover all three aspects of digestion. All three of these products are available without a health coach.

Optimal Measurement Ranges

Optimal pHs According To Breath Rate

Breath Rate	Urine pH	Saliva pH
Above 16	5.8 - 6.3	6.5 - 7.0
Below 16	5.5 - 6.0	6.5 - 7.0

Optimal Blood Pressure Reading
120/80
A systolic number between 112 and 130 is considered to be in range.
A diastolic number between 74 and 87 is considered to be in range.

Optimal Breath Rate
Between 14-18 breaths per minute

Optimal Breath Hold Time
Between 41 - 64 seconds

Continue To Learn

Just like anything, the more you learn, the easier it becomes. Continue learning. Visit our website at www.DoneWithThatBooks.com and soak in piles of free information.

Ask Tony

I can't reply and answer your questions directly, but I can post general answers to people's questions on my website. I have an *Ask Tony* blog where you can submit your questions and I select a question or two to answer each week. Register for our newsletter and we'll send each week's questions and answers to you for free. That way, you can freak your friends out when you know how to improve issues that they're dealing with.

Hidden Chapter

Earlier in this book, I mentioned a "Hidden Chapter" that I placed on my website, www.DoneWithThatBooks.com. I've set it up so you can read this chapter and send it to friends. It can be a good way to introduce your friends to the world of "understanding your own body."

Also, feel free to drop me a line. I'd love to get any feedback, even if that feedback includes cussing. I just like to get mail. I won't be able to answer any questions about your specific chemistry or health issues because there are many laws that prohibit that if you're not a personal client of mine. But if you just bought some ninja socks at the store and want to tell me about it, I'd love to hear from you.

Book Updates

My co-authors and I are constantly learning more about nutrition and how the body really works. Be sure to click on BOOK TOOLS > BOOK UPDATES on www.DoneWithThatBooks.com, and find this book title to read about any findings we have come across since we released this book.

Follow Me

You can find my social fanciness at:

Facebook.com/KickItInTheNuts
Twitter - @KickItInTheNuts

My First Movie

If you're not sick of me yet, go to the site for my documentary, *Why Am I So Fat?*. You can watch trailers and videos, and by the time you read this book, the movie may be out.

www.WhyAmISoFatMovie.com

Facebook.com/FatMovie
Twitter - @SoFatMovie

Join The Community And Get Support

On my movie website you can also join our weight loss community totally FREE. Make friends, share goals and successes and find answers to your questions from people who are losing the weight and keeping it off. Support counts. Get you some.

www.whyamisofatmovie.com/community

Private Facebook Support Group

Find our private support team on Facebook. Click "join group" and your membership will be approved by the admin.

www.facebook.com/groups/kickyourfatsupport

References

To check out references used in this book, go to , www.DoneWithThatBooks.com and click on BOOK TOOLS > REFERENCES.

Be Excited

Right now, in your hand, you are holding answers that some people search for their entire lives and never find. You now have knowledge that can be the "cheat sheet" to your health and your life. Don't take it for granted.

Final Words

For the final words of this book, I select crewneck and spindle.

APPENDIX A

More Digestive Explanations

Reflux, Heartburn And GERD

Now that you understand the benefits of both acid production and bile flow working correctly, let's talk about issues that can pop up when one side is not working optimally. I'm referring to the fiction that is the billion dollar industry of reflux, heartburn, and GERD (gastroesophageal reflux disease). The marketing surrounding these issues may mislead an individual more than just about any other current health information out there. First of all, there are many different causes of reflux; but very few cases, if any, are actually caused by "too much acid," as advertisers explain when marketing their products.

At the bottom of your esophagus, there is a little valve called an LES, or lower esophageal sphincter. This valve opens to let food enter the stomach and then it closes, so that the food doesn't go back up your esophagus and burn you. Sometimes, people have a small hiatal hernia where part of the stomach is pulled up above the diaphragm. This can keep that valve from closing and can result in an acid reflux problem. That is one possibility.

However, the most common cause of reflux problems involves the acid level of the stomach. The LES is actually HCL sensitive, meaning that when the stomach makes enough HCL, it activates that valve to close so digesting food doesn't reflux back up. I've already mentioned that some people don't make enough HCL on their own. So doesn't it make sense that, if there isn't enough HCL in the stomach to trigger the valve, the valve would stay open and they would get reflux? People aren't having reflux because of too much acid; they're having reflux because there is not enough acid.

Pharmaceutical companies sell us drugs that turn the acid off, so that when we experience reflux, we can't feel the burning and we assume the originating issue has been dealt with. The problem with that is twofold. First, the stomach also contains digestive enzymes that can come back up with reflux. These digestive enzymes are made to break down protein. What is the esophagus made of? Yes, protein. Therefore, using these drugs stops the burning sensation, but it doesn't stop all the damage that reflux can cause. A reduction in acid coming up could certainly reduce damage. However, it's important to understand that the enzymes coming back up the esophagus still have the ability to cause damage as well. The second problem created by turning off the acid is... you just turned off the acid. I've already covered how important your stomach acid is, how it is the safety barrier for your entire body and how it's an ignorant idea to turn it off.

When you hear about a drug being a proton pump inhibitor (PPI), this refers to the hydrogen proton pump in the human body. These drugs restrict the body from producing hydrogen. Hydrogen is required for the body to make its own HCL, so by turning off the hydrogen, you turn off the acid. Not only are the proton-pump-inhibitor-type drugs another punch in the mouth to your liver (I already discussed how all drugs work by overwhelming the liver enough to be able to stay in the system and do their job), they also turn off your digestion. Now, any food you eat not only doesn't nourish your body like it is intended to, but also this undigested, rotting, fermenting food becomes another problem for your body to try to remove or to store in fat cells. Pretty good little pill, huh?

To reduce reflux, most reflux sufferers can actually *increase* the amount of stomach acid they have which will trigger the LES to close so they no longer experience reflux. This also allows the body to fully break down its food, pull out the minerals and then use those minerals to make the proper amount of stomach acid. Look forward to reading more about how to improve these issues in *Done With Reflux, Heartburn & GERD*.

Crohn's, Colitis, And IBS

What about the other end of digestion? What about the bile side of the action? If bile is not flowing well enough to neutralize the acid product coming from the stomach, now there is acid going through the intestines. And why does the stomach make acid? The primary job of stomach acid is digesting protein. It's the hydrochloric acid that breaks down food and allows protein to become accessible to the body. Think about it; if you don't neutralize that acid, what do you think it's going to do to your intestines? Your intestines are made out of protein, just like your esophagus. How about that? Does anybody you know have symptoms that were diagnosed as IBS, Crohn's, or colitis? Don't you think this could just be the acid that has been produced in the stomach, that has not been neutralized sufficiently in the duodenum by the proper amount of alkaline bile? Now this acid product goes through the intestines like "Zingo!" Why? Because the acidity of this product is making the intestines burn and the body is going to respond to this acidity and march that product right through the person in a big hurry. With this understanding, doesn't it make sense that it comes shooting out the back door in such a rush?

Beyond that, sodium likes to follow chloride. Water likes to follow sodium. So there's also going to be sodium that is attracted to this chloride in the hydrochloric acid (the hydrochloric acid that didn't get neutralized). Then more water will go to the bowels since chloride from HCL that has not been neutralized will draw the sodium with its water into the bowel. It would be like the boy band One Direction showing up to your cookout because they wanted hot dogs. Not only would you have five less hot dogs, you would also have a yard filled with thousands of screaming little girls. The good news is, the water rushing to this guy's bowels will help dilute this acid product that is burning the intestinal walls. The bad news is, he just messed his pants. This guy is going to have diarrhea and he is going to wonder why, when he sits on the John, it's like he was shot from rockets. It's because his body is saying, "Get this acid product that is burning the daylights out of my little intestines out of here!"

Probiotics and gut flora are a hot topic these days. The people that experience these diarrhea-type issues need help in this arena because that un-neutralized acid scorching through their intestines just fried their gut flora. The terrain needs to be right for gut flora to flourish. As you can imagine, the towering inferno of fire is not the right terrain. This is a very vague explanation, and you will better understand this scenario when I release *Done With Crohn's, Colitis, & IBS,* but it's a great visualization to help explain the balance that is required in order for digestion to function correctly. Both ends of the process are important. It's clear that trouble arises when one side or the other isn't holding up its end of the bargain.

Birth Control Medications

Birth control medications work because they close off the fallopian tubes, preventing the eggs from dropping. Now the woman can't get pregnant, so it works. The problem is, the mechanism in the drug can't tell the difference between a fallopian tube and a gallbladder tube, so it can close the latter off as well. The level at which the gallbladder tube is closed can vary from woman to woman. If the gallbladder tube is shut, bile can't flow correctly and I've already covered how much that can blow.

When bile can't flow correctly, you can't properly digest your food and break it down into its elemental components. You may also get nauseous because bile is the main method that the body uses to remove toxins out the south gate (bowels). If your bile flow reduces because of birth control meds, those toxins can build up and you can experience nausea. It's your body's way of telling you, "Look, we can't handle the food you've put in here, do you really need to keep adding more?"

In addition to turning off the body's main path of junk removal, birth control medications are a synthetic drug. In order for the dose to stay in the body long enough to do its job, it has to be a dose high enough to overwhelm the liver. Otherwise, the liver would just remove it from the body. So, any drug can't work unless it first punches your liver in the mouth. Now, the drug occupies the liver and the liver can't do its normal job of removing toxins. As the toxins get backed up, you get nauseous or you can gain weight since your body is forced to store those toxins in fat cells. That's one of the reasons so many women gain weight on the pill.

Birth control meds are also believed to kill all, or most of, your intestinal flora. If birth control medication stops a woman's bile from flowing correctly, there is nothing to cool off the acid product coming from the stomach and the intestinal flora can burn up. Without the beneficial bacteria, bad guys start to take over, creating an overgrowth of harmful bacteria and yeast, like candida.

Just in case you didn't catch my drift here, birth control medication can be one of the worst things a woman can do if she wants to have a healthy body. I realize pregnancy has the potential to wreak havoc on the body as well; at least with pregnancy, 10 years later you have someone to take out your trash for you. However, there is a freedom of choice in these matters, and there are birth control options available that will allow you to continue digesting your food properly.

Gallbladder Removal/Gallstones/Olive Oil-Lemon Drink

When I see a client with health issue after health issue, one of my first questions is, "Do you still have your gallbladder?" Doctors are taught that the gallbladder really doesn't do anything anyway; so, if there are stones or blockages, why not just yank it out? The problem is that your gallbladder is where your body stores bile, and without the proper amount of bile, you can't digest your food completely. The gallbladder also concentrates the bile and makes it stronger, so that when its alkalinity drops down on the acid product from the stomach, there is a good digestive sizzle. You've already learned how proper digestion is needed to obtain nutrients from your food. Eventually, without proper digestion, all the mineral and nutrient deficiencies will cause problems and even imbalances. The majority of health issues lead back to digestion in one way or another. You can digest food correctly only if you have enough acid in your stomach, enough bile from the gallbladder, and bicarb and enzymes from the pancreas dropping down into your duodenum. Without a gallbladder there is no bile storage, so you rarely have enough bile.

The digestive system is a crazy, complex, miraculous machine. With so many bits and pieces at play, the system is vulnerable to problems that would cause it to function below par. Do you really think a system will work the way it is meant to if you take out part of it (i.e. the gallbladder) and chuck it in the garbage? When any part of the digestive process is not functioning, troubles can show up for months, decades, or even a lifetime. You may not even know you're having digestive concerns because you feel okay when you eat (or you've forgotten what it feels like to feel good). But the lack of nutrients coming into the system, which can be created by a lack of digestion, is always going to come back to bite you in the butt. They may even literally bite you in the butt. (That was a parasite joke for those who didn't keep up.)

There is one technique that can simulate bile production from the gallbladder. Many people who have lost their gallbladder use this technique with success to improve their digestion. You can buy ox bile supplements in most health food stores. However, remember that bile is alkaline. If you take an ox bile product with your food, you're going to neutralize your stomach acid while it's still in your stomach. That's not fun. The trick is to take the ox bile product about two hours after a meal, or at least an hour before a meal. I like the hour before a meal best, but it can be difficult to remember that all the time. By moving that bile through your intestines between your meals, you can neutralize the acid product coming from your stomach and almost simulate the sizzle that all the cool kids have in their digestion. This ox bile really isn't going to work as well as true digestion, but without a gallbladder, this ox bile schedule can be one of the most effective options for any type of improvement.

Many people who have had their gallbladder removed will eventually end up with some type of loose stool issue. Since there isn't enough bile storage to neutralize the acid coming from the stomach, that acid just keeps trucking through the intestinal tract. The hitch is that this issue usually arises months or even years after they've had their gallbladder removed, so they never connect the two events. Using an ox bile product (as I described in the previous paragraph) is the most effective method I know to improve or prevent these loose stool issues, outside of buying a used gallbladder from someone at a garage sale (though I'm not sure how that would work with all the haggling that goes on at garage sales).

If you have gallstones and you're thinking about having your gallbladder removed, you might want to try smashing yourself in the face with a hammer instead. You may indeed prefer a nice hammer smashing over some of the troubles I have seen from people who have had their gallbladder removed. There are things you can do to improve your gallbladder function and help soften those gallstones without cutting out the whole package. If someone told you that your big toe needed to be removed, you would make sure he knew what he was talking about; you would also be careful that you did not get a "second opinion" from some crony of the guy who gave you the first opinion. We know that because of gangrene or something very grievous, some big toes do need to be removed. But if you went into the doctor's office with toenail fungus and the doctor said the answer was to cut off your toe, you would probably find somebody else to help you. It seems a person would value his gallbladder at least as much as his big toe. I think internal organs generally eclipse appendages in value, but that's just me. If doctors were educated on how digestion really works, it would eliminate the billion dollar industry of antacids and acid-stopping drugs. Since doctors are not educated on how digestion works, doesn't it make sense that they view the gallbladder as if it were a disposable Ziploc baggie that can just be dumped in the trash?

There is an old-school remedy for a gallbladder attack that still holds true today. Instructions were even printed right on the label of every carton of epsom salt. The label said, "Take 4 tsp of epsom salt mixed in warm water." This will clear most gallbladder attacks because it can squirt the bile through and clear out the blockage. Be warned that this little trick can give you some crazy diarrhea since epsom salt is magnesium sulfate. Both magnesium and sulfur products can push more water to the bowels, so a large dose of magnesium sulfate can create a bit of a show shooting out the back door. But an episode of diarrhea beats a lifetime of diarrhea every time. You would still need to do the work to get your bile to flow better so you can soften up those stones and keep more stones from forming, but this is a great little trick that has worked for over a hundred years for those suffering from gallbladder attacks.

There are some great recipes on the Internet for olive oil and lemon drinks that can help clear out a gallbladder. However, if you do any cleanses like this that can also clear out a liver, and your bile isn't flowing well, you're just dumping all these toxins into the body while the body has no way to remove them. This can trigger some crazy rashes as a result of the body trying to push junk out through the skin, or you can really overload and hurt your kidneys as they try to handle the whole load. With this in mind, be sure you learn how to thin your bile and get it flowing better with specific beet leaf products before you try any of those liver/gallbladder-type cleanses. They can bring about some big trouble if you don't. Are you listening to me right now? This is important, so please don't ignore what I'm saying and go straight for a heavy duty liver cleanse without first addressing your bile flow with the beet leaf products described in chapter three.

Appendix B

Intermediate Testing Procedures

Here I include procedures for intermediate tests that you can run yourself to acquire more information about your chemistry. You should have already read chapter seven and eight before jumping into these intermediate testing procedures.

To get the most from these intermediate testing procedures, you will need to include the results from your simple self-tests from chapter seven. Be sure to have your filled-in *Data Tracking Sheet* handy so you can include that data along with any new findings from the intermediate tests discussed here. The simple tests from chapter seven include:

- pH of Urine and Saliva
- Blood Pressure
- Breath Rate
- Breath Hold Time
- Blood Glucose

Many of the tests explained in this appendix will not only provide more information about the imbalances discussed in this book, they could also give insight to additional imbalances that were not covered in the main chapters. In Appendix C you will learn about the Sympathetic/Parasympathetic Imbalances, and the Acid/Alkaline Imbalances.

To perform one of these tests, you will need to get a pack of 11-parameter testing strips. You can find these urinalysis reagent test strips on www.NaturalReference.com under the category, Self Monitoring.

If you have acquired the tools needed to run the intermediate tests, go to www.DoneWithThatBooks.com and click BOOK TOOLS to download an *Intermediate Imbalance Guide* to use for these procedures. You will input the information from these procedures onto the *Intermediate Imbalance Guide* instead of the basic version. You will learn how to fill this guide out later in this appendix.

These are great tests that everyone should run initially, if you have the ability to do so. You won't need to run most of these tests as often as you may the frequently used tests from chapter seven, but they can still provide excellent information as you get started.

Resting to Standing - Blood Pressure Test

To get an indication of how your body is recovering from a given stress, you can perform a "resting to standing" blood pressure reading. You will actually take your blood pressure reading two times in a row during this test.

1. To test your resting blood pressure: Lie down and test on your left arm according to the directions for your blood pressure cuff, just like you did previously in your normal resting blood pressure test in chapter seven.
2. To test your standing blood pressure: Remain in a lying position, push the button to start the inflation again, then stand up and hold your arm still as not to disturb the machine from taking its reading. You may need to have the machine in your other hand so you can hold it as still as possible as you get up. If the tube from the cuff to the machine is long enough, setting the machine on a table next to you is the best option. If the tube is not long enough, you will have to try to hold the machine as still as possible (along with holding yourself as still as possible) so the machine will not show an error code and require you to retest. If you do get an error code, you will want to lie back down for about 30 seconds to relax and do both steps one and two again.

Since you won't likely perform this test very often, a space is not reserved for it on the *Data Tracking Sheet*. Instead, just place both resting and standing readings on each line separated by a slash. For example, your systolic pressure line might look like this: 122/130. The 122 would indicate your systolic (top) number while you were lying down and the 130 would represent your systolic number when you were standing up.

Then, you can do the same thing for your diastolic and pulse numbers. The ideal result is to see your standing systolic reading higher than your resting systolic reading. If the standing number is lower, this can be an indication that the system may be having a hard time recovering from a given stress.

Dermographic Line

To perform this test, run the non-ink side of a pen across the inside of your arm and then wait 20-30 seconds to see if your skin turns red, white, or the mark just disappears. If the mark disappears, you would be considered balanced in this test.

This is an autonomic nervous system indicator. Typically if a person's vascular system is constricted, the dermographic line stays with a white center and can indicate the individual is leaning too far on the sympathetic side. If the dermographic line stays red, that can indicate a person is leaning toward the parasympathetic side.

Gag Reflex

Gag reflex is another indicator of the autonomic nervous system. High gag reflex is indicating that a person is leaning toward the parasympathetic side. The lack of a gag reflex indicates a leaning toward the sympathetic side. No test is required here. Simply ask yourself, if I'm brushing my teeth and the toothbrush goes a little too far back, do I have a tendency to gag?

Pupil Size

Pupil size is another indicator of the autonomic nervous system. Small pupils indicate parasympathetic; large pupils indicate sympathetic. Looking at the colored area of your eye, if your pupils cover less than 25% of that space, they can be considered small. If your pupils cover more than 50% of the colored area, they can be considered large. If your pupils take up between 25% - 50% of the colored space, this can be considered normal.

11-Parameter Urine Dipstick

On the website, www.NaturalReference.com, you can find a product, Urispec 11-way urine test strips. A canister of 100 test strips will run you about $45 and very few people will need to order these more than once. The Urispec 11-way urine test strips (also referred to as a 10-parameter urine test strip) measure blood, urobilinogen, bilirubin, protein, nitrite, ketones, ascorbic acid, glucose, pH, specific gravity and leukocytes, in urine. Not only can these measurements help you recognize which imbalances may be the most severe for you, but also, individuals could uncover some fairly major issues that could cause all kinds of trouble if undetected. In my opinion, with these test strips, people can uncover information that is very meaningful—all for about forty five cents a strip.

When using an 11-parameter urine test strip, all of the measurements can be read right away except the leukocytes reading. You want to start a two-minute timer as soon as you dampen the test strip and read the leukocytes box right at that two minute time. Pee into a cup and then dip the strip all the way into the cup. You may have to bend the strip a little by pushing the strip against the bottom of the cup in order to get all the colored boxes covered in urine. Pull the strip out right away and touch its edge on a paper towel to wick away some of the excess urine. Read the colors against the color chart on the strips container. On the *Data Tracking Sheet*, circle the colored boxes that match the colors on your dipstick for each reading.

This dipstick is a great, cheap way to look at some more in-depth numbers. I recommend using this 11-parameter dipstick at least once to get a bigger picture of what is going on with your body. Of course, you'll want to perform repeat tests if the dipstick test indicates a problem that you need to track. As I explain each parameter, understand that some of the words are all big and fancy. I just want to let you know what's available on these dipsticks. In this section, I give you a quick blurb about some of these variables. I don't spend time defining what some of these terms mean. Instead, I just let you know what indications they can provide.

Non-Hemolyzed / Hemolyzed
Blood should not be seen in urine. If it is, that could be an indication of either kidney or bladder distress or trauma. Sometimes non-hemolyzed

blood can be seen during a woman's monthly cycle; if that is the case, the test should be administered again at a different time of the month.

Bilirubin
Bilirubin should not be seen in the urine. When bilirubin is seen in the urine, that means it did not go out the biliary pathway, down through the intestines and out the south gate (your butt). It is a validator that the biliary pathway isn't running as nicely as it should. Since bile flow is so important for digestion and waste removal, this is an excellent parameter to have access to.

Urobilinogen
Urobilinogen is not normally seen in urine. Urobilinogen is bilirubin that has been eaten for lunch in the intestines by bacteria. When bacteria eats bilirubin, they poop urobilinogen. This can be common if an individual is constipated.

Protein
Protein should not be seen in the urine. If it is, that can be an indicator that the kidneys may be overwhelmed. Protein in the urine can also be an indicator that the body is breaking down its own tissue.

Nitrite
A positive reading for nitrite is one of the indicators of a UTI (urinary tract infection)—some type of bacteria in the bladder.

Ketones
Ketones are produced by the burning of fat. Typically diabetics show ketones because they are not burning carbohydrates, they are burning fat. People on the Atkins Diet were given ketone strips to show that they had reached the goal of ketosis, so that they would burn fat. I'm not saying this is your goal. This parameter can help indicate if your body is predisposed to burn more fat or more glucose.

Ascorbic Acid
Ascorbic acid will alter the readings on the dipstick. So while this reading lets you know how much ascorbic acid might be being excreted in the urine, it also alerts you that some of the reagents may react improperly when there is too much ascorbic acid.

Glucose

The dipstick color chart shows that some glucose in the urine is "normal." I might agree that is "common" however one would not want to conclude that it is optimal or "normal." I don't feel it is correct that glucose should be in people's urine. Typically you see a glucose reading in the negative box, showing no glucose—that is how you want to see it.

pH

I already talked about pH in chapter seven. This is just nice to have on the strip so you can conveniently check pH with all the other parameters.

Specific Gravity

Specific gravity can be used to validate whether or not your body is leaning too anabolic or too catabolic. This alone is not an indication, however, it can be a great piece of data when looking for further confirmation.

Leukocytes

If you see both leukocytes and nitrite in the urine, that is a very positive indicator of a urinary tract infection and bacteria in the bladder.

Bonus Test - Hemochromatosis

Hemochromatosis is also known as iron overload. Women who still get their period regularly have a much lower risk of experiencing any iron overload conditions since you bleed out iron every month. All the same, since excessive iron levels can cause so much trouble, it's really smart to know your iron levels before you start to use any iron supplements. You can find out for free by donating blood. When you donate blood to the Red Cross, they will always check your iron levels first to make sure you can afford to give up any iron before they start draining blood out of your arm like a giant mosquito. If your iron is too low, they won't let you donate. They will prick your finger and put a drop of your blood into a little box that will output a number indicating your blood iron levels. Below 12.5, they won't let you donate. It is not likely that your number will exceed 15; but if it does, you may want to have a full iron panel done at a lab. I will provide you with a website where you can order one through the Internet, without a doctor's prescription, since it is used only for educational purposes.

There is a hereditary DNA malfunction, hemochromatosis, which is very common for men of Irish or Scottish descent. I am both Irish and Scottish, yet 23 doctors never figured out that I have hemochromatosis. Even though my iron levels were through the roof, nobody picked up on it. One doctor even asked me if I eat a lot of spinach. I told him no and he simply said, "Good, don't." That was it. Seeing that there is no reasonable drug or expensive procedure to correct hemochromatosis, it simply isn't in a doctor's ongoing education, since that education is most commonly provided by pharmaceutical companies.

Iron issues are not often a problem with weight gain. I simply want to add this information to all of our titles to spread awareness of this problem, especially for males (or females who no longer have a period) who are of Irish or Scottish descent. The medical world has removed the iron panel from most standard blood tests to cut down on costs, but they will add it on your test for free if you ask. You just have to know to ask. This condition is very easily treated if you know it is a problem for you. If you don't know, it can certainly cause a world of trouble and baffle doctor after doctor, run up a six figure medical bill, and flat out be annoying.

In the past, I have used the website www.healthcheckusa.com to order iron panels without a doctor's prescription. You simply buy the test online (it will run you about $60) and they email you a form to take into the lab. You just show up with the form and they draw a blood sample. You'll get your results back in a week or two. You may need a professional to help you interpret them, but the result sheet usually at least indicates if specific numbers are high or low. If your numbers are high, the same website also has a hemochromatosis DNA test you can order to find out if you carry any hemochromatosis genes.

It's all about education. There is now a wide variety of tests that you can order online in this manner. It's very easy to do and most tests are reasonably priced. It really works just like when your doctor sends you to a lab for a test, but in this scenario, the test results are sent to the online company and they send you a copy too (either by mail or email). There is value in consumers having the ability to learn about their own bodies so there are companies that can make this happen without a doctor.

Learn More

To learn more about advanced testing equipment or where you can take courses teaching how to use advanced testing methods, contact us at www.DoneWithThatBooks.com. On this same site, you can also click on BOOK TOOLS > ADVANCED TESTING DETAILS, to read about more tests.

Sorting Out The Data

On the *Intermediate Imbalance Guide,* you see that some items have special symbols next to them. The items with a dagger symbol (†) are measurements that you will need to use the 11-parameter urine dipsticks to acquire. The delta symbol (Δ) indicates measurements acquired with use of a special set of equipment or with help from a professional. You can see that you can gain quite a lot of info with just the basic tests that were outlined in chapter seven, using tools like pH strips, a blood pressure cuff, and a stopwatch or egg timer.

You can follow along as I go through each measurement on the *Intermediate Imbalance Guide.* Many measurements are self-explanatory, but there are a few that I describe in a little more detail because they could use extra clarification. You can then use this as a reference tool as you're filling out your *Intermediate Imbalance Guide.* You don't want to check off an item if you don't really understand what it means. Having blank items is normal and should be expected. You want to check off only the items that are clearly a problem for you. For example, under catabolic, you see "Soft/Loose Stool." Check it off only if that is something you have been experiencing frequently, over the last month or so. Don't just check it off because you went to Mexico once and had some butt soup for two weeks. In that same regard, don't say you're not constipated if you're using two tablespoons of Milk of Magnesia every day in order to see any movement. Check off only the things that are apparent for you regularly so you don't sway your "snapshot" and make yourself look like someone you're not.

Imbalance Guide Content

Symbols Key

< less than (i.e. Pulse < 70 means Pulse is less than 70)
> greater than (i.e. Glucose > 100 means Glucose is greater than 100)
† requires an 11-parameter urine dipsticks
Δ requires special equipment or a professional

Electrolyte Status

For both of these imbalances under "Electrolyte Status," the numbers are pretty self-explanatory. *Resting Systolic BP* is the top number of your blood pressure while you are lying down or resting in a seated position. *Standing Diastolic BP* is the bottom number of your blood pressure while you are in a standing position. *Pulse* is the number that comes up on the very bottom of most automatic blood pressure cuffs (for this form you want to use the pulse from the lying or seated position). Some individuals have a pulse that skips beats. These individuals should understand that this is unacceptable, even though it is often seen by professionals as "normal." It's best to regard a skipping pulse as far from "ideal." This issue can be time sensitive enough to talk to a health professional.

Imbalance - Electrolyte Deficiency

- Low Blood Pressure (Resting Systolic BP < 112)
- Standing Diastalolic BP < 73
- Pulse < 70

Imbalance - Electrolyte Excess

- High Blood Pressure (Resting Systolic BP > 130)
- Standing Diastolic BP > 87

Circadian Rhythm (Cellular Permeability)

Imbalance - Anabolic

- Urine pH > 6.3

- Saliva pH < 6.6
- † Specific Gravity < 1.011
- Low Debris in Urine (This means that if you have your urine in a clear cup, you really won't see much floating around in there. Anabolic people are usually stuck in the rebuilding state, so they're not doing a lot of breaking down of old tissues or cells and the amount of debris found in the urine is much lower. You see the opposite under the catabolic state as a catabolic individual seems to always be peeing out junk the body is throwing away.)
- Hard Stool/Constipation
- High Body Temp
- Polyuria (Polyuria means frequent urination.)
- Difficult to Rise (Meaning the snooze button might be your best friend.)
- Δ Adjusted Surface Tension > 69
- Δ Saliva mS < 4.5
- Δ Urine rH2 High

Imbalance - Catabolic

- Urine pH < 6.1
- Saliva pH > 6.9
- † Specific Gravity > 1.020
- Soft/Loose Stool
- Oliguria (Infrequent urination, or frequent but in small amounts.)
- † Protein on Dipstick (This can be a strong catabolic marker because it's an indication that the body is breaking down tissues in the body. The protein that you're seeing here is protein from bodily tissues and usually not protein from a chicken sandwich.)
- Wake Easily
- Low Body Temp
- High Debris in Urine
- Migraines (A true migraine starts in the back of the head or the neck. The word "migraine" has come to describe any really bad headache, but not all headaches are truly migraines. If your headaches start at the front or top of your head, don't check this item.)
- Δ Adjusted Surface Tension < 67
- Δ Saliva mS > 5.5
- Δ Urine rH2 Low

Energy Production

Imbalance - Carb Burner

- Breath Rate > 18bpm (The "bpm" stands for breaths per minute. Remember, each inhale counts as one. Don't count on both the inhale and the exhale.)
- Breath Hold < 45sec
- Low Blood Pressure (Resting Systolic BP < 112)
- Δ Glucose < 70 (I categorized this in the "need equipment" group, but you could do this test with a glucometer that can be picked up at any pharmacy.)
- Urine pH > 6.3
- Saliva pH < 6.6
- Irritable When Hungry

Imbalance - Fat Burner

- Breath Rate < 14bpm
- Breath Hold > 60sec
- High Blood Pressure (Resting Systolic BP > 133)
- Δ Glucose > 100
- Urine pH < 6.1
- Saliva pH > 6.9
- Type II Diabetes

Autonomic Nervous System

Imbalance - Parasympathetic

- Small Pupils
- Pulse Pressure < 37 (The pulse pressure is a measurement found by subtracting your Resting Diastolic BP number from your Resting Systolic BP number. This number is your pulse pressure. When you register on *The Coalition* and input your blood pressure numbers into the progress charts, the charts will automatically calculate your pulse pressure for you and display it on the graph as well.)
- Gag Reflex Increased (If you brush your teeth and your toothbrush goes a little further back, do you gag? When you go to the dentist, do you gag?)
- Red Dermographic Line (With this test, you run the non-ink, round end of a pen across the inside of your arm and then wait 20-30 seconds to see if your skin turns red, white, or the

mark just disappears. If the mark disappears, you don't need to add a check here. If it turns white, you'll place the check under "White Dermographic Line" in the Sympathetic section.)

- Low Body Temp (Below 98.6 degrees Fahrenheit. It should probably be at least a full point below or above before you would check this box or the high body temp box under sympathetic.)
- Warm Dry Hands
- Fingertips Warmer than Triceps (This is too hard to test on yourself since your triceps are the back of your upper arm, but you can have someone grab your fingertips and your triceps at the same time and tell you which is warmer. I recommend not having someone on the subway help you with this. Awkward.)
- Allergies
- Asthma

Imbalance - Sympathetic

- Large Pupils
- Pulse Pressure > 46
- Gag Reflex Decreased (You generally don't have a gag reflex.)
- White Dermographic Line
- High Body Temp
- Cold Hands
- Fingertips Colder than Triceps

Acid/Alkaline Balance

Imbalance - Tending to Acidosis

- Breath Rate > 18bpm
- Breath Hold < 41sec
- Shortness of Breath

Imbalance - Tending to Alkalosis

- Breath Rate < 14bpm
- Breath Hold > 64sec

- Low Blood Pressure (Resting Systolic BP < 112)
- Standing Diastalolic BP < 73
- Burping or Bloating (Many people don't really understand what bloating means. If you ask a woman, "Do your clothes fit tighter at night than when you put them on in the morning?" and she says, "Yes," she's bloating. As far as burping goes, I'm not talking about a huge belch. But if you have little burps after a meal, that is burping. Many people don't even notice that they burp until you ask them and they'll come back a day later and say, "Ya know, I really do burp.")
- Passing Gas
- Reflux/Heartburn
- Δ Total Ureas < 13
- Light Colored Stool (Either it is lighter than the color of corrugated cardboard, or your stool color will vary from light to dark depending on what you eat.)
- Constipation
- Urgent Diarrhea
- Nausea
- Δ rH2 > 20 or Δ rH2 < 17.5
- † Bilirubin on Dipstick

Okay, I Can Add Check Marks... Now What?

Once you've gone through the *Intermediate Imbalance Guide* and added a check mark next to each piece of information that applies to you, you're ready to begin getting to know yourself. As you look over each imbalance box, the idea is just to see if one side has more check marks than the other side, and by how much. An entire box could have almost no check marks, or the check marks could be evenly distributed to both sides. Either of those options can be an indication of balance in that area. However, if you have more check marks on one side of an imbalance box than you do on the other side, that can be an indication of an area that could use some work. You're going to have to use your judgment here. Having one check mark on one side, and none on the other side, is hardly evidence of an imbalance. I really like to see at least a 30% increase of the check marks on one side compared to the other side before I start to consider there to be any imbalance. Of course, I usually consider measurements to be more influential than symptoms in most cases.

Don't confirm an imbalance with just symptoms. If you have a few symptoms that are common for an imbalance, but none of your numbers point in that direction, I don't usually view that as enough to point me in any one direction. I really want to let the chemistry guide me and then use symptoms as tools of confirmation that the chemistry is an accurate picture. If an imbalance appears to be strong, go to the bottom of the *Intermediate Imbalance Guide* and circle that imbalance. If it looks like you could be leaning that direction, but it's not so bad, you can just underline the imbalance to indicate that it needs work, but may not be your biggest trouble area. While evaluating your numbers, also look at how far out of range your numbers are. For example, if your systolic blood pressure is 89, that's a pretty long way from 112 so you can add more weight to that particular parameter. If your systolic blood pressure is 111, yes, that is still below range, but you may have just caught yourself at a low point and you'll want to test that number a couple more times over the next week or so.

When you test all your numbers, you're really looking at a range. You don't know if the day that you tested is an example of your best day or your worst day. That is why you will continue to check the simple self-tests a couple times a week so you can start to look for patterns in your numbers. If your systolic blood pressure is below 95 every time you test it, you know it's low. Just keep in mind that you're not using NASA equipment. It's just a blood pressure cuff you picked up at the pharmacy. You may often notice that you can check your blood pressure and see a systolic of 101 and then check it a few minutes later and see a systolic of 92. That's okay. Those are both low and you at least understand the range that you are in. It is the same with pH strips. You're using pH strips that are just indicating a measurement that you're interpreting through a color, you're not using a pH meter that's accurate to the hundredth.

Conclusions

Once you've completed this process, make your conclusions just like you did in chapter eight. The only difference is you now have more data to guide your decision making process. In Appendix C you can read more details about all of the imbalances covered in this section.

APPENDIX C

Imbalances

I like to include an explanation of all ten imbalances in the appendix of all of my books. This allows you to use this section as a reference source and gives me the chance to cover any imbalances that may not be covered from book to book. With that in mind, some of this material may be review for you. However, since I didn't cover four of the imbalances in Kick Your Fat in the Nuts, I include explanations of the Sympathetic and Parasympathetic Imbalances, and the Acid and Alkaline Imbalances here.

Electrolyte State

The electrolyte state is defined by blood pressure (though a professional health coach may have equipment that can look at other variables in this equation, like conductivity of urine and saliva). In the world of natural health, where the terrain of the body gives so many insights into how the body is functioning, if an imbalance can exist in one direction, there must be an opposite to that imbalance. Otherwise, there would be no middle ground, no place where the body could be considered "balanced." Seems reasonable, right?

Imbalance - Electrolyte Deficiency

Very few doctors will ever complain about your blood pressure being low. Since there is no drug for low blood pressure, the ramifications are not in their training. We all know that high blood pressure can cause heart attacks and strokes (blowouts). When they say your blood pressure is great even though it's too low, they're saying that you'll never have a blowout. But is it fun to run around on flat tires all day?

An optimal blood pressure reading is said to be 120 over 80. So, if 140 over 90 is considered high blood pressure in the medical world, wouldn't having those numbers off by the same amount in the other direction be regarded as low blood pressure? Shouldn't a reading of 100 over 70 be considered low?

When blood pressure is low, this is often a reflection of low mineral content in the bloodstream. When the mineral levels decrease, it is a reflection of a decrease in your salts or the vascular system being too open (dilated). Our mineral content not only comes from actual salt, but from our food too. If your digestion is not working properly, you can't assimilate the minerals from the food you're eating and the mineral content in the system can decrease. There are a few other possible contributing factors that can result in low blood pressure. In most cases, however, digestion is the most prevalent contributing factor to low blood pressure. When we see low blood pressure, for example, anything lower than a systolic reading (the top number) of 112 and a diastolic reading (the bottom number) lower than 73, we consider that there is likely an Electrolyte Deficiency Imbalance present.

The minerals, or salts, in the system represent the conductivity, or ability for electricity to flow through the system. When the mineral content is low, there's no spark; and energy can be low. Without this energy, the brain can't function at its full potential, a result created by the lack of minerals required for signals to travel through. Many people with depression, and even other manifestations of "mental illness," are often just cases where there is not enough mineral in the system. Low mineral levels often mean there's not enough spark to give the brain what it needs to function correctly, or there is not enough mineral to control blood pH sufficiently.

Possible symptoms that can show up with an Electrolyte Deficiency Imbalance:

- chronic fatigue
- low blood pressure
- menstrual cramps
- poor circulation
- decreased libido
- depression or anxiety
- vertigo or dizziness when standing
- cravings

- insomnia

Imbalance - Electrolyte Excess

If an Electrolyte Deficiency Imbalance normally indicates a lack of electrolytes, the opposite would be a state where too many electrolytes are present. This is called an Electrolyte Excess Imbalance.

In general, high blood pressure can be an expression of insufficient, or lousy, kidney function. This means that, when excessive electrolytes become concentrated in the bodily fluids, it's usually a result of insufficient hydration (not drinking enough clean water) or impaired excretion of mineral salts through the kidneys. High blood pressure can also result from a constricted vascular system. In any case, electrolyte stress can lead to hypertension (high blood pressure) and other circulatory and cardiovascular problems. A vascular system that is constricted often points to an autonomic nervous system issue or a buildup on the arterial walls. (I talk more about the autonomic nervous system when I talk about Sympathetic and Parasympathetic Imbalances later in this appendix.)

Stiffening arterial walls can lift pulse pressure, which is the difference between the systolic and diastolic blood pressure numbers. When the pulse pressure becomes greater and greater as the arterial walls become stiffer and stiffer, the heart becomes weaker and weaker. If you are a person with high blood pressure who is trying to bring it down naturally, watching the pulse pressure correct itself helps to validate that you are doing the right thing. Remember, *The Coalition for Health Education* has a tool that calculates your pulse pressure for you so you can just monitor the changes without worrying about the math or really understanding what pulse pressure is. Possible symptoms that can show up with an Electrolyte Excess Imbalance:
- high blood pressure
- hardening of the arteries
- heart attack
- stroke
- poor circulation
- inability to properly transport oxygen, nutrients, waste products, antibodies and more, throughout your system

Catabolic/Anabolic States

At the cellular level, the body is always in an anabolic or catabolic state, or in the process of switching back and forth between the two. During the day, our cell membranes are intended to open up (much like a flower) so nutrients can get in and out more easily. This "more open" state is called a catabolic state. At night, our cell membranes are intended to become more closed (again, like a flower) so nutrients cannot get in and out as easily. This "more closed" state is called an anabolic state. The anabolic and catabolic states, at the cellular level, are as obvious a fact as day and night on Earth or tides in the ocean. Both states are appropriate, and even necessary, for a body to function optimally. Due to many possible factors, some people can get stuck in one state and their body will not switch back and forth as intended.

Our cells are made up of different types of fats: fatty acids and sterols. If there are too many sterols in the cell membrane, and not enough fatty acids, the body can be predisposed to become stuck in an anabolic state. With too many fatty acids and not enough sterols, we could be predisposed to get stuck in a catabolic state (the opposite of an anabolic state). To make the body operate correctly, we need to oscillate back and forth from the anabolic state at night, while we sleep, and a catabolic state during the day, while we're active. Without this natural oscillation, many problems can occur. When the body shifts from anabolic to catabolic, that's when the endorphins in the brain are released, which can help people from becoming depressed. Though there are many other factors that more commonly contribute to depression, you can see that this natural oscillation between the anabolic and catabolic states can be important.

Imbalance - Anabolic

First of all, there are many benefits that take place while a body is in an anabolic state. This is the state where the body engages in most of its repairing or rebuilding processes. You've probably heard the word anabolic in reference to steroids. Weightlifters take anabolic steroids in order to be in the tissue building, anabolic state when they are not playing fair with muscle building.

While an anabolic state can have its benefits, any state can cause problems when pushed to an extreme. Although it is very appropriate for the cells to be in an anabolic state at night, some individuals will stay in a more anabolic state most of the time. These individuals are said to be experiencing an Anabolic Imbalance.

If you're stuck in an anabolic state most of the time, it can be very hard to get up in the morning because your body, at the cellular level, is actually still in sleep mode. In the same way that many people who suffer from insomnia are stuck in a catabolic state where their body is always awake, anabolic people can have a hard time getting their bodies in motion in the morning. The snooze button can be their best friend. Be sure to understand, however, that everyone who experiences insomnia is not necessarily stuck in a catabolic state. You will soon be able to read more about this topic in *Done With Insomnia*. Just don't think that, if you suffer from insomnia, you must not have an Anabolic Imbalance because a Catabolic Imbalance is only one possible cause for insomnia. There are insomnia cases that exist quite well in an anabolic state too. Also, don't think that if you pop right out of bed in the morning that you can't have an Anabolic Imbalance. Remember, imbalances can show their heads in different ways for different people. There are no "rules" to follow, only guidelines to help you along.

This Anabolic Imbalance can also cause constipation by sending too much of the body's water to the kidneys and not enough to the bowels, making the stool harder and more difficult to move. An Anabolic Imbalance can also cause individuals to pee high volumes of urine frequently throughout the day. They will often have to get up in the middle of the night to tinkle.

Possible symptoms that can show up with an Anabolic Imbalance:
- constipation or hard stool
- tachycardia (rapid heart rate)
- anxiety/panic attacks
- frequent urination
- difficulty waking in the morning
- viral problems

Since an overly anabolic state can be described as a lack of fatty acids at the cellular level, increasing your fatty acid intake can be one method to help improve this imbalance. However, I find that most individuals with this imbalance really need to use more nutrients like specific vitamins, minerals and amino acids, more than fatty acids, in order to see lasting improvement. Increasing your fatty acid intake may be a place to start when attempting to improve an Anabolic Imbalance, but they are not all created equal and taking rancid fatty acid supplements can be more harmful than good. Yes, mainstream media loves to cram the benefits of fatty acids down our throats; but not only are fatty acids not beneficial for some imbalances, rancid fatty acids are not beneficial for anyone.

Beyond buying the right supplements, also be sure not to just assume you have an imbalance because you're experiencing some (or even all) of the symptoms that commonly show up with that imbalance. Without looking at your specific chemistry, and understanding how your body is operating, you're really just throwing darts when you try to treat symptoms that way.

Imbalance - Catabolic

When it comes to cellular permeability, the catabolic state is the opposite of the anabolic state. It's the other side of the coin. The catabolic state is where the body kind of "breaks down and cleans house," so to speak. In a catabolic state, the body is primed to use oxygen to create energy, so it is appropriate to be in a catabolic state during your waking hours to keep you going all day. This, along with what I just explained about the anabolic state, helps to show how both the anabolic and catabolic states are appropriate during the appropriate times. However, in the same way that I talked about people who lean too anabolic, some individuals will stay in a more catabolic state most of the time. These individuals are said to be experiencing a Catabolic Imbalance.

If someone is stuck in a catabolic state, the cell walls are too permeable and this individual will often burn up muscle and protein and even membrane fats. Breaking down tissues and muscle so they can be rebuilt is a beneficial aspect of the catabolic state, but when a person is in that state too often, for too long, that "cleaning house" process can turn into a body that is flat out falling apart. The more muscle we lose, the lower our metabolism, and we may burn less fat.

Insomnia is very common with a Catabolic Imbalance because the cell membranes are more permeable, which is a characteristic of the daytime state. These people can't sleep because their bodies are still awake and operating at full speed. Most sleeping aids will knock you out in the head so you can sleep, but your body will still be wide awake all night. As a result, you might either wake up exhausted or you become tired again a few hours after waking.

Possible symptoms that can show up with a Catabolic Imbalance:
- insomnia
- migraines
- chronic diarrhea or loose stool
- hair falling out
- muscle loss
- chronic pain
- loss of connective tissue or difficulty in healing
- aging quickly
- joint and muscle pain; arthritis (especially rheumatoid)
- oliguria (insufficient urination, perhaps often but in small amounts)
- low body temperature
- bacterial problems

Since an overly catabolic state is sometimes described as a lack of sterols at the cellular level, increasing your intake of sterols and saturated fatty acids, such as real butter or coconut oil, can be one method to help improve this imbalance. However, I find that most individuals with this imbalance also need to use more nutrients like specific vitamins, minerals and amino acids in order to see lasting improvement. That being said, increasing your sterol intake while optimizing digestion can be a great place to start.

Energy Production

The next two imbalances I cover are Fat Burner Imbalance and Carb Burner Imbalance. These deal with energy production and how the body uses food for fuel. Before I explain energy production, understand that I will be leaving out complicated methods the body can use to create energy. They are not important for this explanation.

To create energy, simply speaking, our bodies burn either fat or glucose. Your body is designed to burn both types of fuel for different purposes. Despite that, changes can occur in our bodies, or in our lives, that will train our bodies to prefer one fuel over the other. The body may stop burning the other type of fuel almost entirely. This is another reason why there is no such thing as the diet that is right for everyone. It doesn't exist. Some people burn fats much better than glucose and some people are the opposite. This really puts all these arguments into perspective about "low-carb," "low-fat," "high-protein," "the drunk diet," "I only eat things that start with the letter F..." I could go on for days. They're still all going to be wrong. In order to find the right "diet," you really need to look at a person's biological individuality, because each person processes foods differently.

Imbalance - Carb Burner

Carb Burners are people who are predisposed to burn off all their glucose and do not seem to burn fat very well. Now, it's not that they won't burn fat, but they will always prefer to burn off all their glucose first. This is commonly referred to as hypoglycemic. Just keep in mind that the hypoglycemic can also be a step away from becoming diabetic. "But if he's hypoglycemic, how can he be a step away from becoming diabetic?" It's because many hypoglycemics have way too much insulin in the system and their system responds as though there are five furnaces in the house. Every time the house gets cold, instead of one furnace coming on and slowly warming up the house and then turning off, FIVE furnaces turn on and the house is hot enough to make you cuss by the time the furnaces shut down.

A Carb Burner's insulin can work in this same manner. These individuals have become insulin resistant, but they have not been insulin resistant long enough that the cells have stopped responding to the insulin altogether. They're at that stage where the cells are still responsive enough to the insulin that, when the pancreas produces up to five times the amount of insulin it normally would, it reaches a critical level and all the sugar goes into the cells at one time. These people can get very severe headaches in the front of their heads. They may also complain that their head feels full or they'll get fuzzy brained; this is due to the blood sugar dropping far too rapidly. Using a blood sugar glucometer can quantify that the blood glucose has gone too low. This low blood sugar can make these folks extremely miserable, and being around them when blood sugar levels drop can be equally miserable. If you live with, or if you are this person, you know exactly what I'm talking about.

Possible symptoms that can show up with a Carb Burner Imbalance:
- lack of energy; physical and mental fatigue
- high or low blood sugar
- shortness of breath
- high cholesterol
- overweight or underweight
- irritable when hungry

Imbalance - Fat Burner

If you find that you show indications of having a Fat Burner Imbalance, you most likely are burning much more fat than glucose. If you also have high cholesterol, high triglycerides and a high fasting glucose, any of these markers can be another indication that you are not processing glucose effectively.

Many individuals who are overweight and have this imbalance will ask, "How is it that I'm burning mostly fat but I'm still so fat?" This is because their bodies are turning almost every carb and sugar that they eat into fat. In order to process sugar or glucose, the body is having to take all sugar or glucose coming in and turn it into fat before it is able to be "burned" for energy.

Possible symptoms that can show up with a Fat Burner Imbalance:
- lack of energy; physical and mental fatigue
- Type II Diabetes
- metabolic syndrome (or insulin resistance)
- high blood pressure or cardiovascular disease
- weight gain
- gallbladder trouble

You may have noticed Type II Diabetes on the list above. This doesn't mean that if you have a Fat Burner Imbalance that you're diabetic. It just means that in this fat burning state, the body prefers to burn fat and can often move into a predicament where it will burn very little glucose, if any. In these cases, glucose can accumulate in the bloodstream and, abracadabra, you're diabetic. Remember, I am only describing an imbalance in this section and not a disease. However, a neglected imbalance certainly can manifest itself eventually as a disease, just like neglecting to change the oil in your engine can manifest itself as a blown up engine.

By improving this imbalance and allowing the body to once again process both types of fuel, a person could increase energy and lose some weight, since such a large percentage of glucose would no longer need to be stored as fat.

Autonomic Nervous System

Sympathetic Dominance refers to the autonomic nervous system (ANS). The ANS is a mechanism in the body that happens without having to consciously think about it. You don't have to think about whether your heart is beating, it just does. The other side of the nervous system is the Parasympathetic Dominance.

The sympathetic side is the speed side—the fight or flight response. The parasympathetic side is the slow side—the rest and digest state. These two systems are hard-wired, in a sense, to the heart, the entire digestive system, and all the lower level glands, organs and systems.

Imbalance - Parasympathetic

A Parasympathetic Imbalance is often where I find individuals who suffer from allergies or asthma. This can be a tricky imbalance because if an individual has a strong ANS imbalance, especially on the parasympathetic side, that person can often see a response that is opposite of what is expected when working to balance the body. For example, if a specific food or supplement tends to push one measurement, like urine pH, down for most people, that same food or supplement could actually push up that measurement for a parasympathetic person. I've never heard a good explanation as to why this can occur for some, but it seems the defense system and immunological issues affect this anomaly. It is seen frequently enough in parasympathetics that you need to know this anomaly exists. That is why learning to monitor your body is so important. Monitoring your body will also alert you when the time has come to get the help of a professional who understands the wide variety of nuances that can occur when looking at layer upon layer of imbalances in the body.

Possible symptoms that can show up with a Parasympathetic Imbalance:
  • allergies

- asthma
- small pupil size
- frequent urination
- increased saliva
- muscle cramps at night
- eyes or nose watery
- eyelids swollen
- gag easily
- poor circulation

Imbalance - Sympathetic

The ANS is reactive. As a stress situation presents itself, the system turns on, does its job, and in doing so possibly reaches its outer bounds of homeostasis (perfect balanced health). Thanks to this selfish act of the ANS, other systems in the body can be deprived and suffer. Not unlike the transmission in your car, systems in the body can "lock up" and refuse to shift out of low gear, thus causing a myriad of symptoms such as unpredictable and/or uncalled-for behavior. The stress situations that are instigating the reaction of the ANS could be emotional, nutritional, or mineral in origin. If individuals are stuck in a sympathetic state, they can feel stressed and on edge, and even have trouble sleeping since they are stuck in fight or flight mode.

Possible symptoms that can show up with a Sympathetic Imbalance:
- large pupil size
- low levels of urination
- increased temperature
- sweaty hands
- dry mouth/eyes/nose
- get chills often
- cold extremities (like hands or feet)
- unable to relax
- irritated by strong light

pH Balance - Acid/Alkaline Imbalances

Everybody just calm down. This can be a very hot topic in the world of natural health. If this book is your first taste of natural health, this section may open your eyes to some incredible things. Kind of like the series *LOST*, but this will actually make sense. However, if you have already read, or have been introduced to, information about the pH of the body, I may need to spend time fixing the damage that some other numskulls have created.

The bloodstream has a very narrow pH value that it must stay within in order for our bodies to function properly. If the blood moves too far acid or too far alkaline, we can literally die. The body doesn't want this to happen, so it does whatever it can to keep the bloodstream at a balanced pH level.

In the natural world, when people talk about pH, they frequently talk about how we all need to "alkalize." "Alkalize, alkalize, alkalize." "Alkalize or die a slow, miserable death," they tell us. These pH "gurus" explain how we are all too "acid" and it's killing us one by one. Of course, when someone follows these approaches and tries to alkalize themselves, and they completely fall apart, the guru tells them, "That's okay, you're going through a 'healing crisis'. Just stick to it and you'll be fine." No, what we're going through is a guru crisis. There currently appears to be a crisis where a few gurus need to be punched in the neck so maybe they will stop ruining the well-being of half of their readership.

These readers who started to fall apart after "alkalizing" themselves were likely falling apart because they were pushing an imbalance that already existed even further over the edge. Remember how I talked about the fact that an imbalance can't exist unless there is an equal imbalance in the other direction? If someone told you one pair of glasses will fix everyone's vision, you would question his intelligence or just poke him in the eye. We all know that reading glasses can help farsighted people while nearsighted individuals need the very opposite type of lens. Any author who tells the reader that EVERYONE should do ANYTHING is trying to sell something.

The haphazard confusion starts here; some individuals truly are too "acidic." I talk about what this means in just a moment. For now, I'm going to continue using the same ignorant terminology that most of the pH gurus use. When individuals have an Acid Imbalance, and they truly can benefit from "alkalizing" themselves, these individuals can follow the instructions laid out by a pH guru and they may see tremendous improvement to their health, or at least their well-being. In some cases, these results could even be considered miraculous. Still, let's just calm down for a minute. If we know that every imbalance (like an Acid Imbalance) will have an opposite imbalance in the other direction, what are these pH gurus doing to the people who have an Alkaline Imbalance (the opposite of an Acid Imbalance)? They're making these individuals miserable and calling it a "healing crises," that's what they're doing.

To go right along with all of the pH and alkalizing books and experts out there, we also find shelves upon shelves of "alkalizing" products in every health food store. You can't throw a stick down the aisle of a health food store without hitting a product that boasts its ability to improve your health through alkalizing. (By the way, if you do this, the employees will come right up to you and ask you not to throw sticks in their store anymore... like I'm the one doing something wrong here.) It is also likely that these products will increase in popularity since many people will reap benefits from their use. Many people with an acidity issue, that is. To understand the tragedy in this, let's go over the Acid and Alkaline Imbalances.

The most important thing to understand is that, when I discuss an Acid or Alkaline Imbalance in this series of books, I am talking about blood pH. Measuring urine pH and saliva pH in a context of breath rate and breath hold can be incredibly insightful and useful, but urine pH or saliva pH are not always an indication of the pH of the blood, as many pH gurus will have you believe. It's a nice story, it just happens to be a fictional one. I already showed you how to measure urine pH and saliva pH. For now, I'm just going to dig into blood pH since this is the crucial parameter when looking at an Acid or Alkaline Imbalance.

Imbalance - Tending to Alkalosis

Alkalosis is an imbalance where the bloodstream is too alkaline. When the blood leans alkaline, oxygen can't leave the bloodstream and go to the tissue level where it needs to be to help your body create the energy required to run properly. In science, this is known as the Bohr Effect.

If a doctor checked your oxygen levels, he would put a device called a pulse oximeter on you and he might tell you that your oxygen is great... you have plenty. But, because the bloodstream is too alkaline, the oxygen cannot be released from the bloodstream and go into the tissues where it can be used. The result: You can feel wiped out. The oxygen is there, it just can't get to the right location in order to be properly utilized. In an effort to correct this, when the bloodstream is too alkaline, the body will slow the rate at which you breathe. Carbon dioxide (CO_2) is acid inducing to the bloodstream so the body tries to reduce the amount that you breathe in order to hold on to more CO_2, allowing it to acidify the bloodstream. Pretty neat trick Mother Nature came up with, don't you think? By using the CO_2 to acidify a bloodstream that is too alkaline, some oxygen can be released from the bloodstream and make it to the tissue level.

Possible symptoms that can show up with an Alkaline Imbalance:
- chronic fatigue
- sleep apnea
- joint and muscle pain; arthritis
- allergies; asthma
- muscle cramps
- fluid retention

In regard to sleep apnea, many cases are caused by structural issues (such as a flap that doesn't seem to be flapping correctly), but almost as many are caused by a bloodstream that is too alkaline. The breath rate drops so low due to an overly alkaline bloodstream that eventually the body says, "I'm gonna acidify this bloodstream and get some oxygen down to the tissues where it needs to be even if it kills this guy," and this would show itself as sleep apnea symptoms.

By looking at all the trouble an overly alkaline bloodstream can cause, do you see how important it is to look at people as individuals and measure where they are before you start blabbing about how everyone needs to alkalize? Just because something brings about an amazing result for one person, doesn't mean that it's not going to turn someone else into a zombie. This is another example of how people are different. Why is that so hard for many people to grasp? I've met individuals who can't get enough Maury Povich; yet if you forced me to watch that show, I might not ever talk to you again. We know people are different in their preferences; if they weren't, how would John Tesh have a fan base at all? Since people can have different tastes, doesn't it make sense that they could have different chemistry as well?

The physiology in a person with Acidosis problems expresses too much acid (or H+) in the bloodstream. One cause can be an imbalance in potassium, or an inability of the kidneys to properly excrete the acid and balance is lost. The breath rate in these individuals becomes accelerated because the kidneys, being unable to easily control the acid level in the bloodstream, can be helped by the lungs huffing off CO_2, because CO_2 acidifies the bloodstream. These individuals will normally have a short breath-holding time and a rapid breathing rate, exposing the fact that the kidneys are not having an easy time controlling the pH of the blood. This can be remedied (depending on the cause) by assisting the system to buffer the acids more effectively and excreting them. But this is not just a failure to excrete acids, it's a failure to buffer them. This helps us to understand why using foods or supplements in an effort to "alkalize" an individual can be so beneficial. This is how a pH guru can hit home runs with some people who will then think he is so brilliant. These people with the overly acid issues can really benefit by increasing the nutrients that can be used to buffer these acids. Even a broken clock is right twice a day.

An inability to properly digest protein can often be an issue in these cases since the biggest buffer of acids in the body is protein. Obviously, it is more profitable for the industry to sell green drinks and alkalizing supplements than it is to help people better digest their protein. Yet, in some cases, simply improving protein digestion can be a great step toward giving the body the tools it needs to buffer those acids on its own.

Possible symptoms that can show up with an Acid Imbalance:
- shortness of breath
- rapid heart rate
- allergies
- poor retention of important mineral nutrients
- fluid retention
- poor function of your kidneys, lungs, adrenal glands and many other organs and glands
- digestive issues

Alkalizing Water And Water Filters

The first step in digging through this dung is to remember that some individuals have an Acid Imbalance. Their blood is tending toward being too acid. If this is you, one of these alkalizing water filters could certainly help you feel better if it was pushing your blood to a more balanced state. You would know if it was working or not if your breath rate started to come down. In this scenario, you would start to feel better and would tell all of your friends it was because of the "magic water" that was coming out of your water filter and you're so excited because you only have sixty-three more monthly payments before it is paid off.

Let's not stop there. To a lot of my clients, I will hold up a bottle and say, "Have you heard of this? It's called WATER!" because it's so obvious that they're not drinking any. Water is one of the most important components to our health and yet so few people drink enough to help their bodies wash out all the junk. They think that if they're drinking a soda or coffee, that's enough. "It has water in it," they tell me. But soda and coffee, or even sport drinks, are hardly a replacement for water. None of those beverages have the ability to truly hydrate the cells like water can. Most of those drinks just introduce more junk into the body rather than giving your body what it needs to wash junk out. But tell me this: If a guy pays $3000 for a water filter, do you think he might drink some water? You bet he will! He'll probably go fill up a glass every time he opens his checkbook or checks his bank statement. "Where the heck did all my money go? Oh yeah, I guess I should go get a glass of water."

When you take a person who hasn't been drinking any water, and you start getting H2O down his gullet, that can often be enough to turn his whole world around. You start to hydrate the body, you start to clear out junk. Pounds get dropped, joints become more flexible, all sorts of happy stuff can happen—just by adding some water. Too bad he could have done the same thing with a ninety-nine cent jug of spring water.

I'll call this water filter mortgaging consumer "Bill." Bill tells his friend Tanya about this filter and talks her into buying too. (Certainly this is just about her health and has nothing to do with the fact that Bill will be making money off of Tanya's purchase.) But Tanya starts to feel worse. She's exhausted and finds it easier to just sit on the couch all day. If you checked Tanya's breath rate you might see that it's around eight. With a breath rate that low, it could be that Tanya's blood is leaning too alkaline and this alkalizing water is pushing that imbalance further into the abyss.

Since Tanya hears testimonial after testimonial from people who have improved their health by drinking this water, she thinks it must be something else that is bringing her down. It can't be the water because every multilevel marketing meeting she goes to plays loud music and people dance around because they feel so good. Meanwhile, Tanya's blood is so alkaline that oxygen can't get down to the tissues and she just wants to lay down on the floor until they turn off the Macarena.

When deciding if alkalizing water is right for you, it's crucial to look at breath rate and understand if your blood could benefit from drinking this water or if it's just going to make you worse. Even if you do have an Acid Imbalance, and drinking alkaline water could benefit you, be sure to continue to check your breath rate for improvement. You don't want to correct an Acid Imbalance so well that you create an Alkaline Imbalance. Monitoring yourself and your numbers is what this type of health movement is all about. It's not about finding something that makes you feel better and using that product until you die. It's about using something until your body is balanced and then reducing it until you don't need it anymore.

As a side note, remember that the first thing that water hits is your stomach. If you're drinking alkaline water with your food, that alkalinity is going to reduce the effectiveness of stomach acid levels that may already be too low.

APPENDIX D

Those Who Paved the Way

Dr. Carey Reams

Dr. Carey Reams was an agrarian. He did soil chemistry and he learned, primarily, how to make things grow in the soil. By people coming to him for help, he was pushed into biology and working with animals and humans. What remained at the root of his mentality was all this knowledge about what made produce grow exceptionally well. What needed to be done in order to bring the proper level of minerals into the produce? What got a result in the crop? There are a lot of stories about how Reams adjusted minerals in the soil to affect the growth of produce. If you wanted to do something in soil, he knew how to do it. That mentality was then brought forward into looking at health from a simple ground-up standpoint. Reams looked at the mineral content in a person, much like he looked at the mineral content in the soil.

Dr. Emanuel Revici

Dr. Emanuel Revici was all about looking at the cell's oil-based membrane and the proteins that are mixed in with it. He explained what was going on with the permeability of the cells. Through learning about cellular permeability, we came to understand that there is a natural tide to life, or a rhythm. This is where the anabolic/catabolic language comes into use. We see that during the daytime it is proper for a person to be in a catabolic state—when he is giving his energy to the day. Conversely, as surely as night falls and the dandelion flower closes, the anabolic state is entered and the person goes to sleep to rebuild and restore himself. Everyone needs to be cycling between these two states. As people lose their vitality or resilience, this tide of life becomes impeded and an individual can get stuck in the anabolic or catabolic state 24 hours a day. Without the necessary vitality to allow this natural oscillation process to continue, it is statistically true that those who become stuck in an anabolic state are more prone to viral issues occurring in their system. Those who have lost their resilience and are stuck in a catabolic state are more prone to bacterial issues. Now comes the reasonableness of the system where if a person is really oscillating every evening from catabolic to anabolic, and every morning from anabolic going back to catabolic, then the viruses don't have a home and the bacteria don't have a home because the system is oscillating. There is never a moment when, for many days, there is a hospitable environment for those issues to take hold.

There is a good book about Dr. Revici, written by William Kelley Eidem, called *The Doctor Who Cures Cancer*. This is a story of Revici's life and work and is an excellent introduction into the intellect he provided us.

Thomas Riddick

Thomas Riddick understood colloidal suspensions. What is the bloodstream? It is a colloidal suspension. This is information that painters understand perfectly because, if you can't keep pigment in suspension, then it is going to separate, fall to the bottom of the can and harden. If that pigment falls out of suspension then you aren't going to sell much paint. You aren't going to get the pigment to the wall, it's not going to dry correctly and it isn't going to work. With Riddick's research, we came to understand a lot more about the heart and how to make the bloodstream flow easier so that the heart does not work so hard.

Certainly, when half of America is dying from a heart-related problem, we would be curious to know what to do to make things easier for the heart. That used to be understood before profit-driven thinking took over. I don't want that to sound like I'm bitter, I'm not. I do wish that those who put profit over the public's well-being could be locked in a room and forced to listen to old Menudo albums until they promise to change their ways, but I'm not bitter. I don't want you to think that I'm the type of person that would basically Menudo-style waterboard someone. Still, wouldn't the world be a better place? If this was taken care of, the only issues we would need to get rid of are smoking in public, people who stink, and those that drive slow in the left lane. Order restored.

Dr. Melvin Page

Dr. Melvin Page was a medical doctor whose research showed that proper nutritional balance in the body could not only improve the health of someone's teeth, but also the health of the body would coincide with the improvement of their dental health. He found that, when the calcium-to-phosphorus ratio was in a balanced proportion, the patient would present no cavities. (The actual proportion is ten-to-four in the blood, for those who like it when I say things that make me sound fancy. For those who say, "What the hell is he talking about?" just use the word "balanced.") Moving outside of this ratio would not only present cavities, but other health issues as well.

Dr. Page was also very interested in, and had a lot of success with, hormones. He found that you couldn't even get a good read on hormones if the blood sugar was elevated. For this reason, he would require avoidance of carbohydrates for at least 72 hours before any hormone testing was done. When we look around us today, with the rate that the population is having trouble with diabetes, hypoglycemia, and blood sugar issues, is it any wonder that there are also a lot of hormonal issues going on? Dr. Page had a lot of information that we try to implement.

Dr. Page and all these other doctors serve to validate or challenge each other's views. It's as though they're all looking into the same room (human physiology) but through different windows, giving a different perspective on very similar issues.

Recommended Reading

The Doctor Who Cures Cancer - William Kelley Eidem
The story of Emanuel Revici, M.D. that introduced us to the anabolic/catabolic shifts in the body.

Nutrition and Your Mind - George Watson
An excellent book that demonstrates how the types of foods we eat can make a difference in our physical health <u>and</u> mental health.

MORE ABOUT TONY

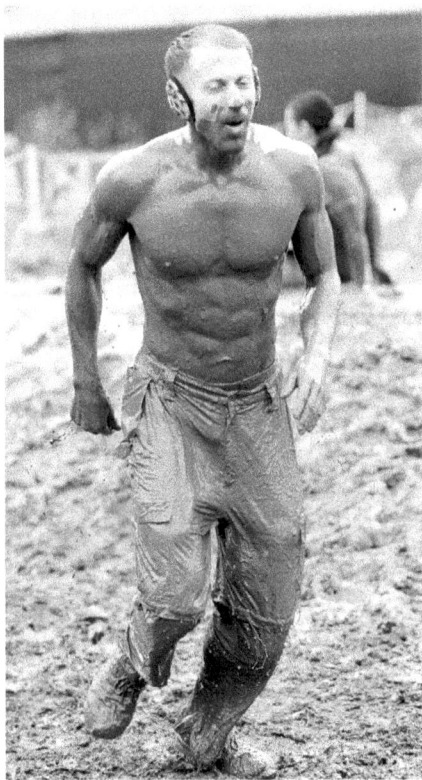

Like most natural health experts, Tony began his career in stand-up comedy. Touring professionally as a comic for nearly a decade, he never envisioned that he would one day teach the world how to sleep, poop, and even lose weight.

On Valentine's Day, 2004, Tony lost his voice and it didn't came back. After twenty-three doctors couldn't figure out the problem, Tony decided it was time to dig for his own answers. Eight years later, not only did Tony figure out his own issues, he also happened upon hidden information about how to improve countless other health problems.

Though Tony likes to boast about the fact that he holds no legitimate credentials (nor does he believe that we need any more "experts" from the same pool of knowledge already failing so many with health issues), he is greatly respected by his peers in the natural health industry. The biggest manufacturers in the health, fitness and organic products industries send Tony their products every year in hopes of winning one of his GearAwards.

 Beyond working with many celebrity clients, Tony is on the executive board of *The Coalition for Health Education*, a nonprofit association that helps professionals and their clients learn about health through nutrition. Additionally, Tony teaches monthly webinars about nutrition to doctors, nutritionists and other health care professionals from more than thirty-five countries.

You can also find Tony producing documentaries like, *Why Am I So Fat?* A film that teaches the truth about weight loss while showcasing Tony's client, Gabe Evans, who lost 200 pounds in 9 ½ months by treating Tony's word as gospel.

To learn more about Tony, visit www.DoneWithThatBooks.com

That's it. Close the book now.